DERMATOLOGY - LABORATORY AND CLINICAL RESEARCH

MYCOSIS FUNGOIDES AND SÉZARY SYNDROME

PATHOGENESIS, DIAGNOSIS AND TREATMENT

DERMATOLOGY - LABORATORY AND CLINICAL RESEARCH

Additional books and e-books in this series can be found on Nova's website under the Series tab.

DERMATOLOGY - LABORATORY AND CLINICAL RESEARCH

MYCOSIS FUNGOIDES AND SÉZARY SYNDROME

PATHOGENESIS, DIAGNOSIS AND TREATMENT

XIAOHUI ZHANG, MD, PHD
AND
LUBOMIR SOKOL, MD, PHD
EDITORS

nova
Medicine & Health
New York

DOI: https://doi.org/10.52305/LFSE9103

NOTICE TO THE READER

Library of Congress Cataloging-in-Publication Data

Names: Zhang, Xiaohui (Associate member of the Department of Pathology), editor. | Sokol, Lubomir, editor.
Title: Mycosis fungoides and sézary syndrome : pathogenesis, diagnosis and treatment / Xiaohui Zhang, MD, PHD, Associate Member, Department of Pathology, H. Lee Moffitt Cancer Center and Research Institute, Tampa, FL, USA, Lubomir Sokol, MD, PHD, Senior member, Department of Malignant Hematology, H. Lee Moffitt Cancer Center and Research Institute, Tampa, FL, USA, editors.
Description: New York : Nova Science Publishers, [2021] | Series: Dermatology - laboratory and clinical research | Includes bibliographical references and index. |
Identifiers: LCCN 2021045863 (print) | LCCN 2021045864 (ebook) | ISBN 9781685070939 (hardcover) | ISBN 9781685071561 (adobe pdf)
Subjects: LCSH: Mycosis fungoides. | Skin--Tumors. | Lymphomas.
Classification: LCC RC280.L9 M93 2021 (print) | LCC RC280.L9 (ebook) | DDC 616.99/477--dc23
LC record available at https://lccn.loc.gov/2021045863
LC ebook record available at https://lccn.loc.gov/2021045864

Published by Nova Science Publishers, Inc. † New York

CONTENTS

Preface

Mycosis fungoides (MF) is the most common subtype of cutaneous lymphomas. The initial diagnosis of MF is often difficult, particularly in the early stage, requiring arduous clinical and pathological workups with repeat skin biopsies. Differential diagnosis ranging from benign dermatoses to other hematolymphoid neoplasms can be tricky and extremely challenging. Clinical management and treatment vary widely among providers and institutions. This book is an up-to-date overview of MF, covering almost every aspect of the disease. The chapters encompass etiology, clinical workup and diagnosis, pathological diagnosis, clinical and pathological variants, differential diagnosis, treatment and prognosis, as well as the state-of-the-art understanding of the molecular genetics of MF. Pediatric MF and Sézary syndrome (SS) are also included for completeness in the book.

In clinical practice, a thorough and insightful book to review the etiopathogenesis, diagnosis, prognosis and treatment of MF is much needed. It is our sincere hope that this book can serve as a practical reference for dermatologists, hematologists, oncologists, general pathologists, dermatopathologists, hematopathologists, and other health care providers treating patients with skin diseases, and clinical researchers interested in MF and SS, and provide guidance on how to diagnose, manage and treat this perplexing disease.

Xiaohui Zhang, MD, PhD
Lubomir Sokol, MD, PhD
Tampa, FL, USA

In: Mycosis Fungoides and Sézary Syndrome ISBN: 978-1-68507-093-9
Editors: X. Zhang and L. Sokol

Chapter 1

EPIDEMIOLOGY AND PATHOGENESIS OF MYCOSIS FUNGOIDES

Rohit Sharma, MD and Xiaohui Zhang**, MD, PhD
Department of Pathology,
H. Lee Moffitt Cancer Center and Research Institute,
Tampa, FL, USA

INTRODUCTION

Cutaneous T-cell lymphomas (CTCLs) are a heterogenous group of lymphoid malignancies derived from skin-homing T cells, accounting for 75-80% of all primary cutaneous lymphomas. Mycosis fungoides (MF) is the most common form of cutaneous lymphoma, accounting for 50-65% of primary cutaneous lymphomas [1]. It is a primary epidermotropic CTCL characterized by infiltrates of small to medium-sized neoplastic T lymphocytes with cerebriform nuclei. Closely related Sézary syndrome (SS) accounts for 5% of CTCL cases. These two types of CTCL have often been grouped together.

* Corresponding Author's Email: Xiaohui.Zhang@moffitt.org.

The term "mycosis fungoides" was coined by French dermatologist Jean-Louis-Marc Alibert in 1806 when he described the clinical presentation of a "mushroom-like fungal disease," which is a misnomer [2]. It was named so because Alibert observed mushroom-like, end stage skin tumors. It is now known that MF is not a fungal infection but rather a type of non-Hodgkin lymphoma. In 1876, Bazin et al. [3] defined the three stages of the disease (patches, plaques, and tumors). Several variants including pagetoid reticulosis (PR), folliculotropic variant and granulomatous variant were described in 1939, 1957, and 1970, respectively [4-6]. SS was named after a French dermatologist Albert Sézary [7], who described this variant of MF in 1938, and has been used for the advanced and erythrodermic form of CTCL characterized by cutaneous and systemic dissemination of neoplastic T cells [8].

In the past decade, the World Health Organization–European Organization for Research and Treatment of Cancer (WHO-EORTC) consensus classification has been a gold standard for the diagnosis and classification of CTCL. This classification was published in 2005 [9, 10] and was updated in the 2008 WHO classification and its 2016 revision (Table 1-1) [11].

Table 1-1. WHO-EORTC classification of MF and its relative frequency and disease-specific survival

WHO-EORTC Classification 2018	Frequency, %*	5-year DSS, %
MF	52	88
MF variants		
Folliculotropic MF	6.7	75
Pagetoid reticulosis	<1	100
Granulomatous slack skin	<1	100
SS	2.7	36

*Percentage of all CTCL cases.

**DSS, disease-specific survival.

EPIDEMIOLOGY

The overall estimated age-adjusted incidence rate of MF is 6.4 per million persons based on Surveillance, Epidemiology and End Results (SEER) registry data from 1973-2002, and 7.7 per million persons in 2001-2005 [12-15]. A consistent increase in incidence has been documented since the 1970s [16]. The incidence of MF is higher in patients of African American descent in comparison to patients of European descent [17]. By race, the incidence was 4.0 for whites, 6.1 for African Americans, 3.0 for Asian/Pacific Islanders, and 0.9 for Native Americans/other/unknown [13]. In this study, non-white populations had significantly different MF incidence rates for different tumor stages compared to whites. The incidence of T0–T2 MF for whites was 3.0 per million compared with 4.0 for African Americans ($p = 0.0015$), 2.4 for Asian/Pacific Islanders ($p = 0.048$), and 0.4 for Native Americans/other/unknown ($p = 0.0023$) [13]. The incidence for T3-T4 MF was 0.5 for whites, 0.9 for African Americans, 0.3 for Asian/Pacific Islanders and 0.6 for Native Americans/other/unknown. Only African Americans apparently had a significant increase in incidence by higher T-stage ($p = 0.0039$). While the age-adjusted incidence rates vary between countries, an increased incidence of MF has been reported in some countries such as Japan [18] and Finland [19]. The age-adjusted incidence rate for SS is 0.1 per million persons [20].

The prevalence of early stage MF in the US is estimated to vary from 5.2 to 6.6 per 100,000 persons [21]. There has been an increase in the prevalence of diagnosed MF and SS. For example, in Finland, the prevalence of MF and SS rose from 2.04 to 5.38 per 100,000, and from 0.16 to 0.36 per 100,000 persons for MF and SS respectively during 1998–2016 [19].

In the United States, the median age of diagnosis of MF is 55 years with men being 1.6 to 2 times more commonly affected than women. The mean age at diagnosis of MF is higher for males than females (58.6 years for males vs. 55.4 for females ($p = 0.0005$)) [13]. Although rarely seen before the age of 30, MF can occur in children and teenagers, constituting 65% of reported pediatric cutaneous lymphoma cases [22]. The prevalence of pediatric MF varies geographically, comprising 4-16% of total MF cases [22-25] (Also see Chapter 7. *Mycosis fungoides in pediatric and adolescent young adult patients*).

The mortality rate from MF is variable and significant survival differences have been demonstrated, which relate to clinical stage. Patients with stage 1 disease demonstrate a mortality rate similar to that of an age-matched control population while those with stage IV disease show a 27% 5-year survival rate and a 10% 15-year survival rate [26]. Table 1.1 shows the relative frequency and survival of 1905 patients with MF, MF variants and SS based on data included in Dutch and Austrian cutaneous lymphoma registries between 2002 and 2017 [27]. Studies have shown that MF has a variable frequency in different geographical regions with less cases in North America in comparison to Europe, ranging from 40% to 90% in different studies conducted in different regions [28]. SS has frequencies ranging from 1% to 15% of CTCL, estimated at 3% globally (95% CI 2% to 4%) [29]. The estimated frequency of the other subtypes of CTCL are depicted in Figure 1-1 [27].

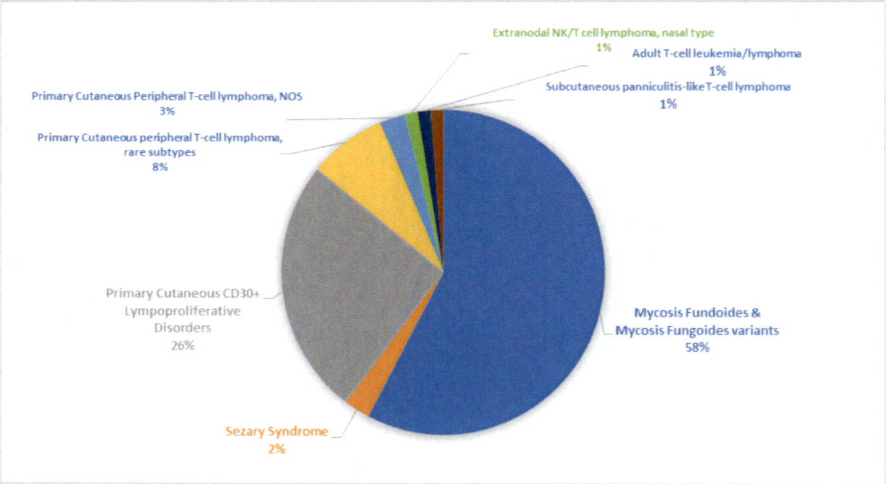

Figure 1-1. Frequency of different subtypes among all cases of CTCL.

ETIOLOGY

The etiology of MF is largely not elucidated, and causative agents/factors have not been clearly defined. Several theories have been suggested, which may contribute to the development and progression of the disease. This has included the involvement of potential infectious agents, occupational factors, ultraviolet light exposure, immunogenetic factors, benign dermatoses, genetic abnormalities, life style and others.

Infectious Agents

Chronic antigenic stimulation via various viruses and/or bacterial infections may contribute to the clonal expasnion and eventual neoplastic tranformation of T cells [30-32]. Many infectious agents are suspected to be associated with MF, including but not limited to *Staphylococcus aureus*, *Borrelia burgdorferi*, Human T-cell leukemia virus type-1 (HTLV-1), and Epstein-Barr Virus (EBV). There have been reports describing MF in patients with HIV infection [33, 34], although this is considered to be rare. See Table 1.2 for other viruses that have been investigated. It has been demonstrated that subjects with multipe infections as oppposed to a single infection have a significantly higher risk for MF [35]. However, the data are limited and the results are controversial with no consistent association between an infectious agent and MF being established [30]. There are possibilities of bystander infections or those that are detected in MF lesions that may not actually contribute to the pathogenesis and evolution of the disease but instead be incidental findings.

Occupational Factors

Few studies have identified geographical clustering of CTCL as a group which may indicate possible unidentified external factors or triggers that are contributing to the development of these diseases in specific regions [36].

The potential for occupational hazards to play a role in development of the disease has also been investigated. Certain occupations have been identifed to have an elevated risk of MF including crop and vegetable farm workers, painters, woodworkers and general carpenters among others. Studies have also suggested that different industrial occupations demonstrate variable associations with the risk of developing MF. Those working as machinists, machine operators, textile workers, construciton workers, foundry operators, wood industry workers, and industrial cleaning service workers are more frequently affected than the others [37].

Ultraviolet Light Exposure

Ultraviolet (UV) light is a known risk factor for the development of melanoma, non-melanomatous skin cancers, and some non-Hodgkin lymphomas. However, regarding the role of UV light in MF development, studies actually have shown a complex picture. A European case–control study observed a link between MF and occupational sun exposure [38]. In line with this, a whole genome and exome sequencing study demonstrated the presence of mutational signatures (high frequency of transitional mutations (C to T) which are associated with UV light exposure in the skin lesions of MF [39]. In contrast, a study based on US SEER data found no association between UV ambient radiation and the risk of MF [40]. In the meantime, a study using the SEER-18 and the National Solar Radiation Database demonstrated that residence in high-UV light exposure areas was associated with up to a 30% lower incidence of MF [41], echoing the underlying mechanisms of skin-directed therapeutic use of UV light in MF patients, in which the UV light can induce lymphotoxicity within the dermis and epidermis, suppressing antigen presenting Langerhans cells, and decreasing malignant CD4+ T lymphocytes. The observations that MF is more common in African Americans than in whites also suggested UV light exposure may have an inhibiting effect for cutaneous T cell malignant transformation. It is probable that combinatorial effects of UV light on skin, including both the immune modulatory effect and mutational impact on skin-resident T-cells, play a complex role in the MF development and pathogenesis.

Immunogenetic Factors

Familial cases have been reported and a study showed that histocompatibility antigens HLA-B8, AW3 and AW31 were more frequent in patients with MF [42]. The potential role of immunogenetics has also been demonstrated with several studies showing an association between specific HLA alleles (HLA-A*24, A*68, A*69, B*35 and DQB1*05:02) and an increased susceptibility of developing MF. In addition, an association between specific HLA alleles and the clinical course of the disease has been identified, relating to long-lasting remission (HLAA*24 and HLA-A*25), frequent relapse (HLA-DRB1*01, DQA1*01:01, DQB1*05:01) and death (HLA-A*68, HLA-B*08, HLA-B*35, HLA-C*03) [43].

Benign Dermatoses

It has been reported that patients with psoriasis and atopic dermatitis, which are known to have familial inheritance, are at a higher risk for MF/SS [44, 45]. Patients with chronic dermatitis [46], or parapsoriasis en plauqes [47, 48] can evolve/progress to MF, with recent molecular evidence that the two (specifically large plaque parapsoriasis and MF) have striking similarities [48]. Another study suggested that many patients had histories of rashes prior to the diagnosis of MF, mainly nonspecific rashes or dermatitis [37]. Some benign inflammatory dermatoses appear to be risk factors for MF, however since differentiation between benign dermatoses from MF could be challenging, this needs to be examined more closely in the future with more advanced molecular techniques as used in the study [48], to differentiate the diseases more precisely and to further elucidate the evolution process if any.

Genetics

There is evidence suggesting a family history of multiple myeloma could pose a risk for developing MF and familial MF cases have been reported [9, 49, 50]. A family history of benign dermatoses appeared to be a risk factor for MF as well [51]. However, there is overall a lack of strong scientific evidence of hereditary susceptibility of CTCL [52] and no inheritable germline mutations have been identified. Nevertheless, MF/SS have diverse and complex genetic abnormalities. Most MF patients have one or more chromosomal abnormalities, such as the loss or gain of genetic material. These genetic abnormalities usually are acquired during the patient's lifetime, rather than inherited. Recurrent chromosomal changes were observed in chromosomes 1, 2, 7, 9, 17, and 19, and the most commonly seen were gain of chromosome regions 1p36, 7, 9q34, 17q24-qter, 19, and loss of 2q36-qter, 9p21, and 17p [53]. Whole-exome/genome NGS and array comparative genomic hybridization studies revealed multiple alterations in various pathways, including the cell cycle and DNA damage repair, JAK-STAT signaling, TCR/NF-κB signaling, chromatin-modifying genes, and MAPK pathway [54, 55] (see Chapter 8. *Molecular genetic updates of mycosis fungoides*).

Life Style

An increase risk has been associated with a smoking history of 40 years or longer, and daily consumption of more than 24 g of alcohol [56].

Other Risk Factors

There is a long list of risk factors that have been investigated, and a summary is listed in Table 1-2 [57].

Table 1-2. Risk factors for MF/SS

Risk factors	Disease	Relative risk	References
Pollutants air exposure and chemicals	MF, SS		[58]
Contaminated water supply, air pollution, or industrial exposure (oil refineries), inciting infectious, radioactive, or chemical agent exposure	MF, SS		[36, 59-61]
Sulphur mustard (SM)	MF		[62]
Agent Orange	MF		[63]
Hydrochlorothiazide (HCTZ)	MF, SS		[58, 64]
History of cigarette smoking ≥ 40years Body mass index ≥ 30 kg/m^2 Moderate leisure time physical activity History of eczema Occupation as painter Occupation as woodworker Occupation as general carpenter Occupation as crop or vegetable farmer	MF, SS	OR = 1.55, 95% CI = 1.04 to 2.31 OR = 1.57, 95% CI = 1.03 to 2.40 OR = 0.46, 95% CI = 0.22 to 0.97 OR = 8.49, 95% CI = 3.31 to 21.80 OR = 3.71, 95% CI = 1.94 to 7.07 OR = 2.20, 95% CI = 1.18 to 4.08 OR = 4.07, 95% CI = 1.54 to 10.75 OR = 2.37, 95% CI = 1.14 to 4.92	[60]
Alcohol use	MF	OR=3.02, 95% CI = 1.34 to 6.79	[56]
High population/dermatologists' density	CTCL,MF		[65, 66]
Family history of atopy	MF	RR = 4.50, 95% CI = 0.89 to 12.95	[51]
Family history of multiple myeloma	MF, SS	OR = 8.49, 95% CI = 3.31 to 21.80	[9, 60]
Common viral/environmental exposure in cases of familial clustering and in married couples	MF		[50, 67-69]

Table 1.2. (Continued)

Risk factors	Disease	Relative risk	References
Genetic susceptibility (Human leukocyte class II antigen DRB1*11)	MF, SS	HLA-DR5- odds ratio OR = 3.62, 1.9 < OR < 10 in MF and OR = 3, 0.9 < OR < 9.3 in SS, HLA-DQB1*03 alleles - OR = 2.15, 1 < OR < 4.5 in MF and OR = 4.7, 1.4 < OR < 5 in SS	[50, 70-72]
Multiple infectious agents	MF		[31, 35, 73]
Human T-cell leukemia/lymphotropic virus type 1 (HTLV-I)	MF		[74-79]
HTLV-II	MF		[74, 80]
Human-immunodeficiency-virus (HIV) infection	CTCL, MF		[81-83]
Human Herpesvirus (HHV) 8	MF		[84, 85]
Epstein-Barr virus	MF, SS		[86-97]
Cytomegalovirus	MF, SS		[98, 99]
Human Herpesvirus (HHV) HHV-6 and HHV-7	MF, SS,		[84, 96, 100, 101]
HHV-8	MF		[85]
Staphylococcus aureus	SS		[102-104]
Chlamydophila pneumoniae	MF, SS		[105, 106]

Pathogenesis

Cell of Origin

A subset (30%) of healthy T lymphocytes have a propensity to home to the skin, typically expressing cutaneous lymphocyte antigen (CLA) and C-C chemokine receptor type 4 and 10 (CCR4 and CCR10) [107]. These cells normally participate in homeostatic immune surveillance of the skin and respond to injury and inflammation of the skin. Malignant T cells in MF are believed to originate from skin homing T cells. T cells that have been isolated from MF lesions on the skin have been shown to express CLA and CCR4, a phenotype that consistent with skin resident effector memory T helper cells [108]. This phenotype differs from that of T-cells in Sézary syndrome in which the cells express CCR7 typically expressed by central memory T cells. The MF malignant T cells are CLA+/CCR4+/L-selectin-/CCR7- (skin resident memory T cell, T_{RM}), whereas the malignant T cells in SS are CLA+/CCR4+/L-selectin+/CCR7+ (skin-tropic central memory T cell, T_{CM}) [108].

In addition, high levels of CCR4 and CCR10 ligands, such as chemokines CCL17, CCL22, and CCL27, produced by keratinocytes and vascular endothelial cells, have been demonstrated within the skin lesions of MF [109, 110], supporting the skin-homing cell as the origin of MF cells, the skin milieu also playing a role in attracting these cells.

Malignant Transformation

Complex chromosomal and molecular abnormalities have been identified, and have been better studied in SS. Most MF/SS driver mutations are copy number alterations (CNA), instead of single nucleotide variants (SNV) [52, 54, 111, 112]. There is a high incidence of complex chromosomal changes which may be related to chromosomal instability [113]. The genetic abnormalities revealed by molecular profiling studies are complex and include genes involved in multiple molecular signaling pathways, which are described in Chapter 8 (Table 8.1, in Chapter 8 *Molecular genetic updates of mycosis fungoides*). For example, *TP53* mutations and *CDKN2A* deletions were significantly enriched in patients with large cell transformation, suggesting their association with disease progression [114]. The affected pathways are broadly involved in T cell activation, function, migration and differentiation.

Immunogenesis

Malignant T cells in MF/SS show a persistent state of activation, which is evidenced by the constitutive phosphorylation of Stat3 [115]. The activated cells have the capacity to produce cytokines, such as interleukin 4, 5 and/or 13 (IL-4, IL-5, IL-13), resulting in a Th2 cytokine profile [116]. A skew from Th1 toward Th2 phenotype in advanced stages of MF/SS can lead to Th1 immunity suppression. Depletion of the healthy lymphocytes caused by the proliferation of the malignant T cells also contributes to the immune suppresion. This Th2 dominance contributes to disease progression through production of IL-4, IL-5 and IL-10, by circumventing the host cell-mediated anti-tumor immune reponse [117]. This can also cause increased risk of secondary infection or malignancy.

Conclusion

MF and SS are lymphoid malignancies derived from skin-homing T cells. There is a trend of increasing incidence for these diseases. The causative etiology of MF is not defined, however, infectious agents, occupational factors, UV light exposure, immunogenetic factors, antecedent benign dermatoses, genetic abnormalities, life style and others are considered to be the risk factors for MF and SS. The MF/SS malignant cells are believed to originate from skin homing T cells. Various chromosomal and molecular abnormalities have been identified and driver mutations are involved in multiple molecular pathways. In addition, Th1 immune suppression and Th2 dominance contribute to disease progression. Elucidating the mechanisms underlying MF/SS development and progression has potential preventative and therapeutic implications.

REFERENCES

[1] Willemze, R., et al., WHO-EORTC classification for cutaneous lymphomas. *Blood*, 2005. 105(10): p. 3768-85.

[2] Mahalingam, M. and V. B. Reddy, Mycosis Fungoides, Then and Now... Have We Travelled? *Adv Anat Pa*thol, 2015. 22(6): p. 376-83.

[3] Bazin, P. A. E., Maladies de la Peau Observees a l'Hopital St. Louis. 1876, Paris.

[4] Zelger, B., et al., Syringotropic cutaneous T-cell lymphoma: a variant of mycosis fungoides? *Br J Dermatol*, 1994. 130(6): p. 765-9.

[5] Fraser-Andrews, E., R. Ashton, and R. Russell-Jones, Pilotropic mycosis fungoides presenting with multiple cysts, comedones and alopecia. *Br J Dermatol*, 1999. 140(1): p. 141-4.

[6] Dabski, K. and H. L. Stoll, Jr., Granulomatous reactions in mycosis fungoides. *J Surg Oncol*, 1987. 34(4): p. 217-29.

[7] Willemze, R., et al., Diagnostic criteria in Sézary's syndrome: a multiparameter study of peripheral blood lymphocytes in 32 patients with erythroderma. *J Invest Dermatol*, 1983. 81(5): p. 392-7.

[8] Swerdlow, S. H., International Agency for Research on Cancer., and World Health Organization., WHO classification of tumours of haematopoietic and lymphoid tissues. 4th ed. *World Health Organization classification of tumours.* 2008, Lyon, France: International Agency for Research on Cancer.

[9] Aschebrook-Kilfoy, B., et al., Medical history, lifestyle, family history, and occupational risk factors for mycosis fungoides and Sézary syndrome: the InterLymph Non-Hodgkin Lymphoma Subtypes Project. *J Natl Cancer Inst Monogr*, 2014. 2014(48): p. 98-105.

[10] LeBoit, P. E., et al., *World Health Organization Classification of Tumours: Pathology and Genetics of Skin Tumours*. 2006., Lyon, France: IARC Press.

[11] SH, S., et al., *World Health Organization Classification of Tumours of Hematopoietic and Lymphoid Tissue.* Revised 4th ed. ed. 2017, Lyon, France: IARC Press.

[12] Korgavkar, K., M. Xiong, and M. Weinstock, Changing incidence trends of cutaneous T-cell lymphoma. *JAMA Dermatol*, 2013. 149(11): p. 1295-9.

[13] Wilson, L. D., G. A. Hinds, and J. B. Yu, Age, race, sex, stage, and incidence of cutaneous lymphoma. *Clin Lymphoma Myeloma Leuk*, 2012. 12(5): p. 291-6.

[14] Bradford, P. T., et al., Cutaneous lymphoma incidence patterns in the United States: a population-based study of 3884 cases. *Blood*, 2009. 113(21): p. 5064-73.

[15] Vonderheid, E. C., et al., Update on erythrodermic cutaneous T-cell lymphoma: report of the International Society for Cutaneous Lymphomas. *J Am Acad Dermatol,* 2002. 46(1): p. 95-106.

[16] Wilcox, R. A., Cutaneous T-cell lymphoma: 2016 update on diagnosis, risk-stratification, and management. *Am J Hematol*, 2016. 91(1): p. 151-65.

[17] Geskin, L. J., et al., Cutaneous T-Cell Lymphoma (Mycosis Fungoides and Sézary Syndrome), in *Williams Hematology*, 10e. 2021, McGraw-Hill Education: New York, NY.

[18] Ishihara, K., et al., Statistical profiles of malignant melanoma and other skin cancers in Japan: 2007 update. *Int J Clin Oncol*, 2008. 13(1): p. 33-41.

[19] Keto, J., et al., Mycosis fungoides and Sézary syndrome: a population-wide study on prevalence and health care use in Finland in 1998-2016. *BMC Health Serv Res*, 2021. 21(1): p. 166.

[20] Imam, M. H., et al., Incidence and survival patterns of cutaneous T-cell lymphomas in the United States. *Leuk Lymphoma*, 2013. 54(4): p. 752-9.

[21] Maguire, A., et al., Early-stage Mycosis Fungoides: Epidemiology and Prognosis. *Acta Derm Venereol*, 2020. 100(1): p. adv00013.

[22] Wu, J. H., B. A. Cohen, and R. J. Sweren, Mycosis fungoides in pediatric patients: Clinical features, diagnostic challenges, and advances in therapeutic management. *Pediatric dermatology*, 2020. 37(1): p. 18-28.

[23] Fink-Puches, R., et al., The spectrum of cutaneous lymphomas in patients less than 20 years of age. *Pediatric dermatology*, 2004. 21(5): p. 525-533.

[24] Nanda, A., et al., Mycosis fungoides in Arab children and adolescents: a report of 36 patients from Kuwait. *Pediatric Dermatology*, 2010. 27(6): p. 607-613.

[25] Tan, E., Y. K. Tay, and Y. C. Giam, Profile and outcome of childhood mycosis fungoides in Singapore. *Pediatric dermatology*, 2000. 17(5): p. 352-356.

[26] Kim, Y. H., et al., Long-term outcome of 525 patients with mycosis fungoides and Sézary syndrome: clinical prognostic factors and risk for disease progression. *Arch Dermatol*, 2003. 139(7): p. 857-66.

[27] Willemze, R., et al., The 2018 update of the WHO-EORTC classification for primary cutaneous lymphomas. *Blood,* 2019. 133(16): p. 1703-1714.

[28] Dobos, G., et al., Epidemiology of Cutaneous T-Cell Lymphomas: A Systematic Review and Meta-Analysis of 16,953 Patients. *Cancers* (Basel), 2020. 12(10).

[29] Jenni, D., et al., Primary cutaneous lymphoma: two-decade comparison in a population of 263 cases from a Swiss tertiary referral centre. *Br J Dermatol*, 2011. 164(5): p. 1071-7.

[30] Mirvish, J. J., et al., Role of infectious agents in cutaneous T-cell lymphoma: facts and controversies. *Clin Dermatol*, 2013. 31(4): p. 423-431.

[31] Tan, R. S., et al., Mycosis fungoides--a disease of antigen persistence. *Br J Dermatol*, 1974. 91(6): p. 607-16.

[32] Wohl, Y. and E. Tur, Environmental risk factors for mycosis fungoides. *Curr Probl Dermatol*, 2007. 35: p. 52-64.

[33] Munoz-Perez, M. A., et al., Cutaneous T-cell lymphoma and human immunodeficiency virus infection: 2 cases and a review of the literature. *Acta Derm Venereol*, 1999. 79(2): p. 153-5.

[34] Nahass, G. T., C. A. Kraffert, and N. S. Penneys, Cutaneous T-cell lymphoma associated with the acquired immunodeficiency syndrome. *Arch Dermatol*, 1991. 127(7): p. 1020-2.

[35] Bonin, S., et al., Evidence of multiple infectious agents in mycosis fungoides lesions. *Exp Mol Pathol*, 2010. 89(1): p. 46-50.

[36] Litvinov, I. V., et al., Identification of geographic clustering and regions spared by cutaneous T-cell lymphoma in Texas using 2 distinct cancer registries. *Cancer*, 2015. 121(12): p. 1993-2003.

[37] Cohen, S. R., et al., Clinicopathologic relationships, survival, and therapy in 59 patients with observations on occupation as a new prognostic factor. *Cancer,* 1980. 46(12): p. 2654-66.

[38] Morales-Suarez-Varela, M. M., et al., Occupational sun exposure and mycosis fungoides: a European multicenter case-control study. *J Occup Environ Med,* 2006. 48(4): p. 390-3.

[39] Jones, C. L., et al., Spectrum of mutational signatures in T-cell lymphoma reveals a key role for UV radiation in cutaneous T-cell lymphoma. *Sci Rep*, 2021. 11(1): p. 3962.

[40] Cahoon, E. K., et al., Relationship between ambient ultraviolet radiation and non-Hodgkin lymphoma subtypes: a U.S. population-based study of racial and ethnic groups. *Int J Cancer*, 2015. 136(5): p. E432-41.

[41] DeStefano, C. B., et al., The impact of environmental ultraviolet exposure on the clinical course of mycosis fungoides. *J Am Acad Dermatol,* 2019. 81(5): p. 1074-1077.

[42] Schneider, B. F., et al., Familial occurrence of cutaneous T cell lymphoma: a case report of monozygotic twin sisters. *Leukemia,* 1995. 9(11): p. 1979-81.

[43] Brazzelli, V., et al., Immunogenetic factors in mycosis fungoides: can the HLA system influence the susceptibility and prognosis of the disease? Long-term follow-up study of 46 patients. *J Eur Acad Dermatol Venereol*, 2014. 28(12): p. 1732-7.

[44] Gelfand, J. M., et al., The risk of lymphoma in patients with psoriasis. *J Invest Dermatol*, 2006. 126(10): p. 2194-201.

[45] Legendre, L., et al., Risk of lymphoma in patients with atopic dermatitis and the role of topical treatment: A systematic review and meta-analysis. *J Am Acad Dermatol*, 2015. 72(6): p. 992-1002.

[46] Fransway, A. F. and R. K. Winkelmann, Chronic dermatitis evolving to mycosis fungoides: report of four cases and review of the literature. *Cutis*, 1988. 41(5): p. 330-5.

[47] Vakeva, L., et al., A retrospective study of the probability of the evolution of parapsoriasis en plaques into mycosis fungoides. *Acta Derm Venereol*, 2005. 85(4): p. 318-23.

[48] Gug, G. and C. Solovan, From Benign Inflammatory Dermatosis to Cutaneous Lymphoma. DNA Copy Number Imbalances in Mycosis Fungoides versus Large Plaque Parapsoriasis. *Medicina* (Kaunas), 2021. 57(5).

[49] Morales-Suárez-Varela, M. M., et al., Occupational risk factors for mycosis fungoides: a European multicenter case-control study. *J Occup Environ Med*, 2004. 46(3): p. 205-11.

[50] Hodak, E., et al., Familial mycosis fungoides: report of 6 kindreds and a study of the HLA system. *J Am Acad Dermatol*, 2005. 52(3 Pt 1): p. 393-402.

[51] Tuyp, E., et al., A case-control study of possible causative factors in mycosis fungoides. *Arch Dermatol*, 1987. 123(2): p. 196-200.

[52] Choi, J., et al., Genomic landscape of cutaneous T cell lymphoma. *Nat Genet*, 2015. 47(9): p. 1011-9.

[53] Prochazkova, M., et al., Common chromosomal abnormalities in mycosis fungoides transformation. Genes Chromosomes *Cancer,* 2007. 46(9): p. 828-38.

[54] da Silva Almeida, A. C., et al., The mutational landscape of cutaneous T cell lymphoma and Sézary syndrome. *Nat Genet*, 2015. 47(12): p. 1465-70.

[55] McGirt, L. Y., et al., Whole-genome sequencing reveals oncogenic mutations in mycosis fungoides. *Blood,* 2015. 126(4): p. 508-19.

[56] Morales Suarez-Varela, M. M., et al., Are alcohol intake and smoking associated with mycosis fungoides? A European multicentre case-control study. *Eur J Cancer*, 2001. 37(3): p. 392-7.

[57] Ghazawi, F. M., et al., Environmental and Other Extrinsic Risk Factors Contributing to the Pathogenesis of Cutaneous T Cell Lymphoma (CTCL). *Front Oncol*, 2019. 9: p. 300.

[58] Fischmann, A. B., et al., Exposure to chemicals, physical agents, and biologic agents in mycosis fungoides and the Sézary syndrome. *Cancer Treat Rep,* 1979. 63(4): p. 591-6.

[59] Litvinov, I. V., et al., Demographic patterns of cutaneous T-cell lymphoma incidence in Texas based on two different cancer registries. *Cancer Med*, 2015. 4(9): p. 1440-7.

[60] Phan, A., R. Veldman, and M. J. Lechowicz, T-cell Lymphoma Epidemiology: the Known and Unknown. *Curr Hematol Malig Rep*, 2016. 11(6): p. 492-503.

[61] Ghazawi, F. M., et al., Comprehensive analysis of cutaneous T-cell lymphoma (CTCL) incidence and mortality in Canada reveals changing trends and geographic clustering for this malignancy. *Cancer,* 2017. 123(18): p. 3550-3567.

[62] Emadi, S. N., et al., Mycosis fungoides two decades after exposure to sulphur mustard: a follow-up of 1100 victims. *J Eur Acad Dermatol Venereol*, 2017. 31(3): p. 432-437.

[63] Jang, M. S., et al., Clinicopathological features of mycosis fungoides in patients exposed to Agent Orange during the Vietnam War. *J Dermatol,* 2013. 40(8): p. 606-12.

[64] Jahan-Tigh, R. R., et al., Hydrochlorothiazide and cutaneous T cell lymphoma: prospective analysis and case series. *Cancer*, 2013. 119(4): p. 825-31.

[65] Moreau, J. F., et al., Non-random geographic distribution of patients with cutaneous T-cell lymphoma in the Greater Pittsburgh Area. *Dermatol Online J,* 2014. 20(7).

[66] Weinstock, M. A. and B. Gardstein, Twenty-year trends in the reported incidence of mycosis fungoides and associated mortality. *Am J Public Health,* 1999. 89(8): p. 1240-4.

[67] Dupin, M., et al., [Conjugal mycosis fungoides]. *Ann Dermatol Venereol,* 1995. 122(9): p. 595-8.

[68] Schmidt, A. N., et al., Conjugal transformed mycosis fungoides: the unknown role of viral infection and environmental exposures in the development of cutaneous T-cell lymphoma. *J Am Acad Dermatol*, 2006. 54(5 Suppl): p. S202-5.

[69] Lozano, A. and M. Duvic, Cutaneous T-cell lymphoma in non-blood-related family members: report of an additional case. *J Am Acad Dermatol,* 2007. 56(3): p. 521.

[70] Jackow, C. M., et al., HLA-DR5 and DQB1*03 class II alleles are associated with cutaneous T-cell lymphoma. *J Invest Dermatol,* 1996. 107(3): p. 373-6.

[71] Safai, B., et al., Association of HLA-DR5 with mycosis fungoides. *J Invest Dermatol*, 1983. 80(5): p. 395-7.

[72] Detmar, M., et al., A case of classical mycosis fungoides associated with human T-cell lymphotropic virus type I. *Br J Dermatol*, 1991. 124(2): p. 198-202.

[73] Linnemann, T., et al., Polyclonal expansion of T cells with the TCR V beta type of the tumour cell in lesions of cutaneous T-cell lymphoma: evidence for possible superantigen involvement. *Br J Dermatol,* 2004. 150(5): p. 1013-7.

[74] Zucker-Franklin, D., W. C. Hooper, and B. L. Evatt, Human lymphotropic retroviruses associated with mycosis fungoides: evidence that human T-cell lymphotropic virus type II (HTLV-II) as well as HTLV-I may play a role in the disease. *Blood,* 1992. 80(6): p. 1537-45.

[75] Pancake, B. A., D. Zucker-Franklin, and E. E. Coutavas, The cutaneous T cell lymphoma, mycosis fungoides, is a human T cell lymphotropic virus-associated disease. A study of 50 patients. *J Clin Invest,* 1995. 95(2): p. 547-54.

[76] Pancake, B. A., E. H. Wassef, and D. Zucker-Franklin, Demonstration of antibodies to human T-cell lymphotropic virus-I tax in patients with the cutaneous T-cell lymphoma, mycosis fungoides, who are

seronegative for antibodies to the structural proteins of the virus. *Blood,* 1996. 88(8): p. 3004-9.

[77] Khan, Z. M., M. Sebenik, and D. Zucker-Franklin, Localization of human T-cell lymphotropic virus-1 tax proviral sequences in skin biopsies of patients with mycosis fungoides by in situ polymerase chain reaction. *J Invest Dermatol*, 1996. 106(4): p. 667-72.

[78] Hall, W. W., et al., Deleted HTLV-I provirus in blood and cutaneous lesions of patients with mycosis fungoides. *Science,* 1991. 253(5017): p. 317-20.

[79] Shohat, M., et al., Evidence for the cofactor role of human T-cell lymphotropic virus type 1 in mycosis fungoides and Sézary syndrome. *Br J Dermatol*, 1999. 141(1): p. 44-9.

[80] Poiesz, B., et al., HTLV-II-associated cutaneous T-cell lymphoma in a patient with HIV-1 infection. *N Engl J Med*, 2000. 342(13): p. 930-6.

[81] Bachelez, H., F. Hadida, and G. Gorochov, Massive infiltration of the skin by HIV-specific cytotoxic $CD8^+$ T cells. *N Engl J Med*, 1996. 335(1): p. 61-2.

[82] Wilkins, K., et al., Cutaneous malignancy and human immunodeficiency virus disease. *J Am Acad Dermatol*, 2006. 54(2): p. 189-206; quiz 207-10.

[83] Biggar, R. J., et al., Risk of T-cell lymphomas in persons with AIDS. *J Acquir Immune Defic Syndr*, 2001. 26(4): p. 371-6.

[84] Erkek, E., et al., Identification of herpes simplex virus DNA and lack of human herpesvirus-8 DNA in mycosis fungoides. *Acta Derm Venereol,* 2002. 82(3): p. 214-6.

[85] Kreuter, A., et al., High association of human herpesvirus 8 in large-plaque parapsoriasis and mycosis fungoides. *Arch Dermatol*, 2008. 144(8): p. 1011-6.

[86] Lee, P. Y., et al., Possible role of Epstein-Barr virus infection in cutaneous T-cell lymphomas. *J Invest Dermatol*, 1990. 95(3): p. 309-12.

[87] Jumbou, O., et al., Increased anti-Epstein-Barr virus antibodies in epidermotropic cutaneous T-cell lymphoma: a study of 64 patients. *Br J Dermatol*, 1997. 136(2): p. 212-6.

[88] Park, S., et al., Primary cutaneous Epstein-Barr virus-associated T-cell lymphoproliferative disorder-2 cases with unusual, prolonged clinical course. *Am J Dermatopathol*, 2010. 32(8): p. 832-6.

[89] Borisch, B., et al., Recurrent cutaneous anaplastic large cell (CD30+) lymphoma associated with Epstein-Barr virus. A case report with 9-year follow-up. *Am J Surg Pathol*, 1992. 16(8): p. 796-801.

[90] Mouly, F., et al., [Aggressive cutaneous T-cell lymphoma associated with the presence of Epstein-Barr virus. 2 cases]. *Ann Dermatol Venereol,* 1996. 123(9): p. 574-6.

[91] Cho, K. H., et al., An Epstein-Barr virus-associated lymphoproliferative lesion of the skin presenting as recurrent necrotic papulovesicles of the face. *Br J Dermatol*, 1996. 134(4): p. 791-6.

[92] Tournadre, A., et al., Cutaneous lymphoma associated with Epstein-Barr virus infection in 2 patients treated with methotrexate. *Mayo Clin Proc*, 2001. 76(8): p. 845-8.

[93] Novelli, M., et al., Epstein-Barr virus in cutaneous T-cell lymphomas: evaluation of the viral presence and significance in skin and peripheral blood. *J Invest Dermatol*, 2009. 129(6): p. 1556-61.

[94] Noorali, S., et al., Prevalence of mycosis fungoides and its association with EBV and HTLV-1 in Pakistanian patients. *Pathol Oncol Res,* 2002. 8(3): p. 194-9.

[95] Dreno, B., et al., Presence of Epstein-Barr virus in cutaneous lesions of mycosis fungoides and Sézary syndrome. *Acta Derm Venereol*, 1994. 74(5): p. 355-7.

[96] Nagore, E., et al., Detection of Epstein-Barr virus and human herpesvirus 7 and 8 genomes in primary cutaneous T- and B-cell lymphomas. *Br J Dermatol,* 2000. 143(2): p. 320-3.

[97] Jumbou, O., et al., [Epstein-Barr virus research by in situ hybridization in 65 cutaneous T cell epidermotropic lymphomas]. *Ann Dermatol Venereol*, 1998. 125(2): p. 90-3.

[98] Herne, K. L., et al., Cytomegalovirus seropositivity is significantly associated with mycosis fungoides and Sézary syndrome. *Blood*, 2003. 101(6): p. 2132-6.

[99] Ballanger, F., et al., Cytomegalovirus: its potential role in the development of cutaneous T-cell lymphoma. *Exp Dermatol*, 2009. 18(6): p. 574-6.

[100] Brice, S. L., et al., Examination of cutaneous T-cell lymphoma for human herpesviruses by using the polymerase chain reaction. *J Cutan Pathol,* 1993. 20(4): p. 304-7.

[101] Ponti, R., et al., Human herpesvirus 7 detection by quantitative real time polymerase chain reaction in primary cutaneous T-cell lymphomas and healthy subjects: lack of a pathogenic role. *Br J Dermatol*, 2008. 159(5): p. 1131-7.

[102] Tokura, Y., et al., Cutaneous colonization with staphylococci influences the disease activity of Sézary syndrome: a potential role for bacterial superantigens. *Br J Dermatol*, 1995. 133(1): p. 6-12.

[103] Tokura, Y., et al., Stimulation of cutaneous T-cell lymphoma cells with superantigenic staphylococcal toxins. *J Invest Dermatol*, 1992. 98(1): p. 33-7.

[104] Sidoti, F., et al., Prevalence and significance of human parvovirus variants in skin from primary cutaneous T cell lymphomas, inflammatory dermatoses and healthy subjects. *Arch Dermatol Res*, 2009. 301(9): p. 647-52.

[105] Abrams, J. T., B. J. Balin, and E. C. Vonderheid, Association between Sézary T cell-activating factor, Chlamydia pneumoniae, and cutaneous T cell lymphoma. *Ann N Y Acad Sci*, 2001. 941: p. 69-85.

[106] Abrams, J. T., et al., Sézary T-cell activating factor is a Chlamydia pneumoniae-associated protein. *Clin Diagn Lab Immunol*, 1999. 6(6): p. 895-905.

[107] Hwang, S. T., Mechanisms of T-cell homing to skin. *Adv Dermatol*, 2001. 17: p. 211-41.

[108] Campbell, J. J., et al., Sézary syndrome and mycosis fungoides arise from distinct T-cell subsets: a biologic rationale for their distinct clinical behaviors. *Blood,* 2010. 116(5): p. 767-71.

[109] Reiss, Y., et al., CC chemokine receptor (CCR)4 and the CCR10 ligand cutaneous T cell-attracting chemokine (CTACK) in lymphocyte trafficking to inflamed skin. *J Exp Med*, 2001. 194(10): p. 1541-7.

[110] Campbell, J. J., et al., The chemokine receptor CCR4 in vascular recognition by cutaneous but not intestinal memory T cells. *Nature,* 1999. 400(6746): p. 776-80.

[111] Ungewickell, A., et al., Genomic analysis of mycosis fungoides and Sézary syndrome identifies recurrent alterations in TNFR2. *Nat Genet*, 2015. 47(9): p. 1056-60.

[112] Damsky, W. E. and J. Choi, Genetics of Cutaneous T Cell Lymphoma: From Bench to Bedside. *Curr Treat Options Oncol*, 2016. 17(7): p. 33.

[113] Larocca, C. and T. Kupper, Mycosis Fungoides and Sézary Syndrome: An Update. *Hematol Oncol Clin North Am*, 2019. 33(1): p. 103-120.

[114] Wang, L., et al., Genomic profiling of Sézary syndrome identifies alterations of key T cell signaling and differentiation genes. *Nat Genet,* 2015. 47(12): p. 1426-34.

[115] Eriksen, K. W., et al., Constitutive STAT3-activation in Sézary syndrome: tyrphostin AG490 inhibits STAT3-activation, interleukin-2 receptor expression and growth of leukemic Sézary cells. *Leukemia*, 2001. 15(5): p. 787-93.

[116] Saed, G., et al., Mycosis fungoides exhibits a Th1-type cell-mediated cytokine profile whereas Sézary syndrome expresses a Th2-type profile. *J Invest Dermatol*, 1994. 103(1): p. 29-33.

[117] Kim, E. J., et al., Immunopathogenesis and therapy of cutaneous T cell lymphoma. *J Clin Invest*, 2005. 115(4): p. 798-812.

In: Mycosis Fungoides and Sézary Syndrome ISBN: 978-1-68507-093-9
Editors: X. Zhang and L. Sokol

Chapter 2

CLINICAL FEATURES AND DIAGNOSTIC WORKUP OF MYCOSIS FUNGOIDES

Grace Wei, Jaclyn Abraham and Lucia Seminario-Vidal*, MD, PhD
Department of Cutaneous Oncology,
H. Lee Moffitt Cancer Center and Research Institute, Tampa, FL, USA

INTRODUCTION

The clinical features of mycosis fungoides (MF) may present similarly to a wide array of dermatoses. Given the propensity of MF to mimic, or conversely be masked by, other cutaneous conditions, many have deemed MF as “the greater imitator” [1, 2]. This section will consider the classical findings on the clinical presentation of mycosis fungoides (MF) and delve into the diagnostic workup needed to effectively and promptly diagnose this challenging condition.

---

* Corresponding Author’s Email: luciasem@usf.edu.

MF typically occurs in the adult population over the age of 50, but children and adolescents are also susceptible to the disease [3]. Epidemiologically, MF is twice as common in males compared to females, with the disease being particularly common amongst patients of color. MF develops in various stages, which includes patch, plaque, and tumor stages, although progression to the tumor stage and extracutaneous involvement is often not observed in patients with early MF [3].

Clinical Features

The classic presentation of MF are well-defined, generalized or localized erythematous scaly patches that are variable in size (Fig. 3-1) [3]. A patch is a lesion of any size that shows little to no elevation compared to the unaffected surrounding skin [4]. It is possible for a patch to show a very small amount of atrophy [5]. Further, these patches may be pruritic in nature and will typically emerge on areas of the body that receive infrequent exposure to sunlight, such as the lower-trunk, breasts, groin, and buttocks [3].

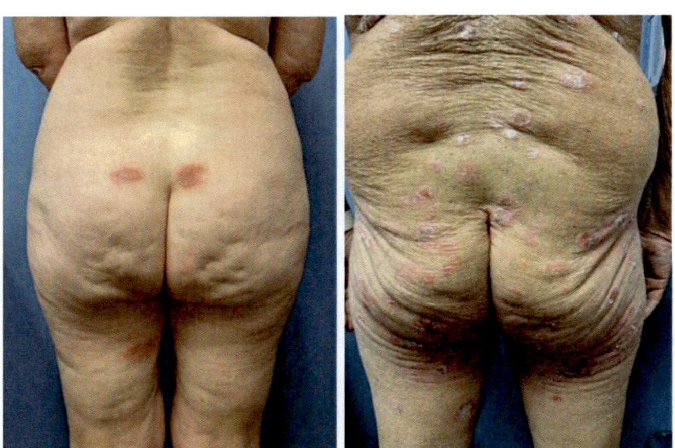

Figure 3-1. Patches: multiple erythematous, scaly, and slightly atrophic lesions, along the posterior buttocks, and back.

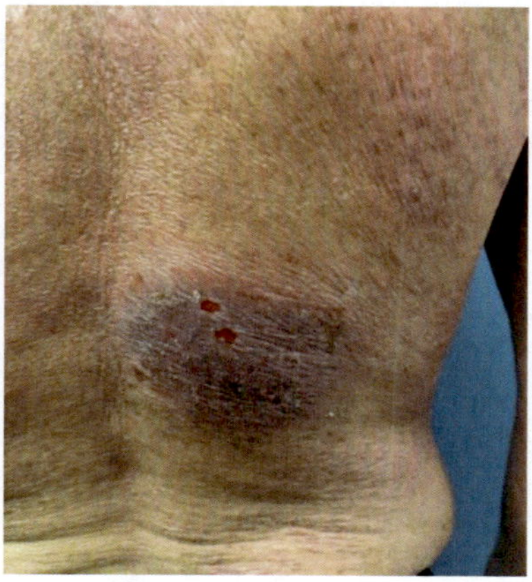

Figure 3-2. Plaque: thick, raised, palpable dry lesion on the back.

Patches can present congruently to plaques, which are elevated lesions of variable size that appear with induration [4]. Plaques may be erythematous with variable scaling and infiltration or can emerge as lesions that are reddish-brown in color (Fig. 3-2) [3]. The lesions may be annular or take on the appearance of a horse-shoe shape, are often raised with well-defined edges, and can distribute asymmetrically on the body, face, or scalp [5].

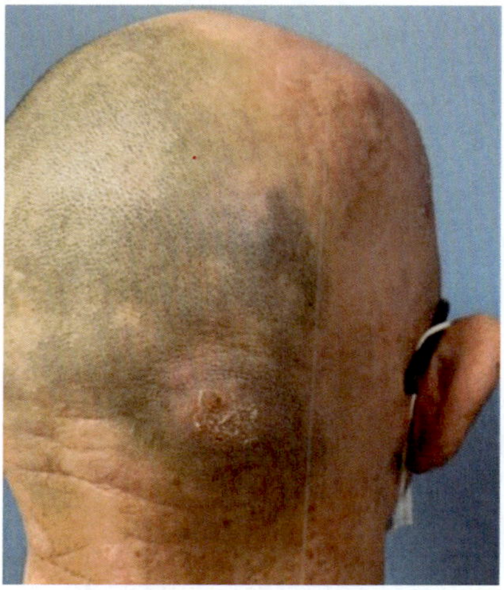

Figure 3-3. Tumor: indurated nodular lesion on the occipital scalp.

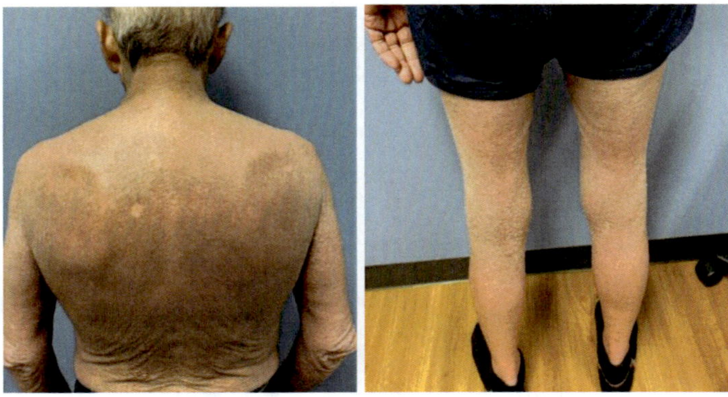

Figure 3-4. Erythroderma: erythema and scaling affecting the majority of the cutaneous surface on the back and posterior thighs and legs.

The tumor stage of MF may appear as erythematous, purple-colored nodules or masses and can arise in combination with patches, plaques or neither (Fig. 3-3) [3, 5]. Tumors are categorized as any solid mass or nodular lesion with a diameter of at least 1 cm, along with evident infiltration or vertical growth into the underlying tissue [4]. Tumors may range in their rate of growth, with some proliferating rapidly while others may remain stagnant [3]. Mucosal involvement is not common but can arise in more advanced stages of the disease [3]. Tumors are prone to ulceration or may eventually show partial regression [3]. It is also possible for MF to cause the development of erythroderma (Fig. 3-4), which should be distinguished from Sézary Syndrome.

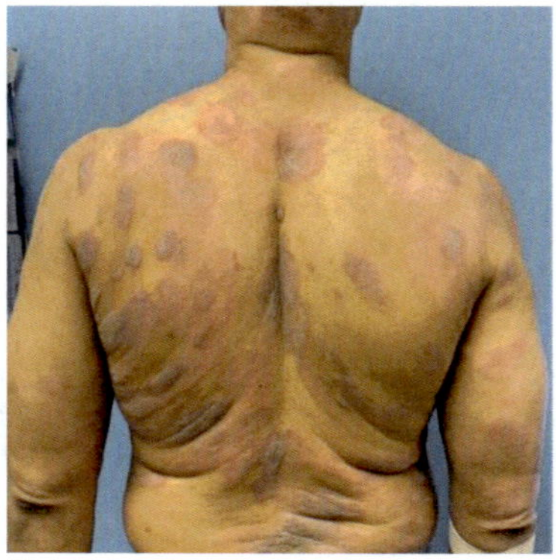

Figure 3-5. Plaques in a patient with a darker skin tone appear to have a greyish hue.

Recent literature has emphasized the disparities that exist between the clinical presentation and prognoses of MF patients attributed to the color of their skin [6, 7]. One study showed that black patients were three times as likely to be diagnosed with MF at a later stage compared to their white counterparts. Further, black male patients tended to present with a higher BSA involvement (19%) and a greater odds-ratio of late stage disease compared to white patients. Black female patients also had an earlier age at both diagnosis and death compared to white patients [6]. Given the disparities that currently exist in MF patients of color, it is crucial to consider how MF may present differently on darker skin tones. For instance, patches and plaques tend to appear less erythematous in darker skin tones, in addition to appearing more greyish-silver in color as opposed to the reddish-brown color observed on lighter skin tones (Fig. 3-5).

Diagnostic Workup

The diagnosis of MF can pose a challenging task, as early stages of the disease often present similarly to more common inflammatory cutaneous conditions, including eczema, psoriasis, and lichenoid dermatoses [8]. This heterogeneic clinical appearance of MF may lead to missed or delayed diagnosis, particularly in early stages, and ultimately result in poorer patient outcomes [9]. Thus, a judicious application of key diagnostic tools is necessary to ensure prompt recognition of MF [3].

Diagnostic Tools

The first component essential for MF diagnosis is a biopsy of suspicious skin lesions. Biopsy sites are carefully identified, often selecting the most indurated regions and avoiding seborrheic lesions or necrotic areas [5, 10]. Further, due to variability in the clinical and histological presentation of MF, it may be necessary to obtain biopsies from multiple sites [11]. Both shave and punch biopsies may be employed, usually, they are obtained in combination. A wide shave biopsy extending to the upper reticular dermis that simultaneously captures a comprehensive region of the dermal-epidermal junction is often preferred [12]. These wide shave biopsies provide greater visualization of the MF dermatopathological architectural infiltrate, a broader area for immunohistochemical staining, and larger amounts of DNA for molecular analysis [12]. Punch biopsies are helpful to differentiate from other dermatoses and to investigate for follicular involvement.

Following biopsy of suspicious lesions, tissue specimens are fixed, processed, sectioned, stained, and mounted for light microscopy analysis [13]. Thus, the second crucial tool for MF diagnosis involves having an expert dermatopathologist that specializes in CTCL perform a detailed review of all tissue slides, including review of at least one paraffin block illustrative of the malignant lesion. In addition to skin biopsy with expert pathological review, the third component essential for MF diagnosis is immunohistochemistry (IHC) staining for CD2, CD3, CD4, CD5, CD7, CD8, CD20, and CD30. Immunophenotyping for MF typically reveals α/β memory T-helper cells with CD2+, CD3+, CD4+, CD5+, CD7-, CD8−, and CD20- markers [5, 14, 15]. Expression of CD30 on MF clonal lymphocytes is variable and more frequently observed in the plaque stage, tumor stage, or in large cell transformations [14]. Notably, loss of CD7 is commonly observed in early stages of MF [8, 16, 17]. However, loss of CD7 is considered non-specific, as it can also occur in other inflammatory skin diseases and should be interpreted in the context of other diagnostic findings [8, 16, 17]. Sufficient diagnostic sensitivity and specificity of loss of CD7 in early patch stage MF requires greater than 90% of T-lymphocytes with a CD7 negative immunophenotype [18].

Finally, molecular analysis of T-cell receptor (TCR) gene rearrangements are also fundamental tool for MF diagnosis. TCR gene rearrangement is a necessary process in T-cell ontogeny involving recombination of the variable, diversity, and joining regions of TCR genes; clonal TCR gene rearrangements are frequently observed in MF, particularly TCR-γ [16, 19, 20]. The sensitivity and specificity of clonal TCR gene rearrangements are variable, with greater sensitivity observed among gene rearrangements analyzed via polymerase chain reaction (PCR) and greater specificity using high-throughput next-generation sequencing [16, 21]. Importantly, however, TCR gene rearrangements may also be observed in benign dermatoses, and thus should be evaluated in aggregate with other MF diagnostic tools [22].

Additional tools may also be situationally employed to supplement the diagnosis of MF in certain circumstances. In select cases, biopsy of lymph nodes or suspicious extracutaneous sites may also be informative if prior skin biopsies were inconclusive, particularly if lymphadenopathy is observed on physical examination or if abnormal lymph node activity is observed on positron emission tomography (PET)/computed tomography (CT) imaging. In these instances, a biopsy of the lymph node is performed in order to facilitate a thorough assessment of tumorous infiltration, whereas use of fine needle aspirates are not recommended [10]. An expanded IHC panel of the following markers may also be performed in indeterminate cases: CD25, CD56, TIA1, granzyme B, TCR-beta, TCR-delta, CXCL13, ICOS, PD-1 [14, 23-27]. Further, use of flow cytometry or a Sézary cell preparation (peripheral blood smear) may be utilized to evaluate the presence of Sézary cells in peripheral blood. Because of the subjective nature of cell counting in a Sézary cell preparation, flow cytometry is generally preferred; further, flow cytometry is also able to detect cellular phenotypic anomalies [28]. Lastly, evaluation of human T-cell lymphotropic virus (HTLV) in the setting of MF suspicion may also be considered. HTLV-1 is a known causative agent in the development of adult T-cell leukemia/lymphoma (ATLL); due to the patches and plaques observed in ATLL bearing striking resemblance to those in MF, a connection between HTLV-1 and MF has been highly debated [29]. While the relationship remains uncertain, assessment of HTLV serology is beneficial in guiding differential diagnoses and thus in guiding therapeutic strategies. Serological testing may be more strongly indicated among patient populations from endemic regions such as Caribbean islands and subjects who are at high-risk for HTLV-1 infection, with proposed risk factors including intravenous drug use, vertical transmission from infected mothers, and sexual transmission

[30]. Importantly, HTLV serology alone is not sufficient for diagnosis of ATLL.

New and Emerging Tools

Recent years have seen a promising surge in new and emerging diagnostic tools for MF. Innovations in biomarker discovery suggest encouraging improvements in the landscape of MF diagnoses are on the rise, such as the TH-1 and TH-2 markers, T-bet and GATA-3, and thymocyte selection-associated high-mobility group box (TOX) [31, 32]. T-bet expression has been shown to have marked elevation in patch stage MF, compared to marginal GATA-3 expression [31]. Similarly, aberrant expression of TOX in MF has also been observed, found to be expressed in over 50% of neoplastic tumor cells in 83% of MF patients, particularly in the CD4+ CD8- immunophenotype [32]. Importantly, while TOX is not limited to MF tumors and it alone is insufficient for diagnostic certainty, it may provide an adjunctive benefit in the diagnosis of MF when combined with other diagnostic tools [32, 33].

The tumor microenvironment and surrounding milieu has also been identified as a target for MF diagnostic advancements, including cellular populations, CD8+ T-lymphocytes, CD1a-positive Langerhans cells, and M2-like macrophages, and cellular proteins, FOXP3 and CCR4. Notably, increased levels of CD8+ T-lymphocytes and Langerhans cells have been shown to correlate with improved survival rates, suggesting a potential role in anti-tumor function and host immune defense [34, 35]. Conversely, M2-like tumor-associated macrophages, a cell population implicated in a number of various cancer types, have been linked to the progression of tumorigenesis and angiogenesis in MF in-vivo mouse models [36]. A key player in the tumor environment of MF are regulatory T-cells (Treg), however the exact role that Tregs play in MF remain ambiguous. Studies have suggested that tumor milieus containing FOXP3, a unique marker and master regulator of Tregs, are associated with improved MF survival [37]. However, others indicate downregulation of Tregs via monoclonal antibody targeting of CCR4 also reduces CCR4+ malignant T-lymphocytes [38].

The expression of therapeutic targets in MF has also greatly expanded in recent years and has been linked to opportunities for diagnostic application in this chronic disease, including expression of CD52, CD30, CD25, CD158a/KIR3DL2, CCR4, PD1/PDL1, CD2, and CD5 [39-44]. Further, emerging prognostic factors, including Ki-67, c-Myc, and Twist, may offer an improved means to identify MF patients with advanced disease early on in their presentation [45]. Markedly increased Ki-67 expression rates have been observed in MF populations with large-cell transformations (LCT), whereas elevated levels of c-Myc and Twist have been observed in advanced stage MF lesions [46, 47].

Limitations

Diagnostic limitations in variability of IHC results in the same patient and/or lesion as well as technical pitfalls of IHC. Studies suggest that nearly one-third of IHCs may be insufficient for diagnostic use, and may result from weak signals, false negative or positive staining, and poor signal-to-noise ratios [48]. Additional constraints include lack of standardized guidelines and limited reproducibility due to variability in tissue preparation and staining, scoring, quality control, and assay optimization [49].

Workup

Key workup components are needed to supplement the essential aforementioned diagnostic tools utilized in identifying MF. First, a comprehensive history and physical exam should be taken for each patient. In addition to a thorough total body skin examination evaluating the type, extent, location, and ulceration of skin lesions, calculations of the percentage of total body surface area (TBSA) and modified severity-weighted assessment tool (mSWAT) should be completed. Hand or palm surface areas are commonly used to estimate TBSA involvement. The generally accepted assumption is that palm plus fingers of the patient roughly represent approximately 1% of TBSA; some studies suggest 1% may be a slight overestimate for adults and underestimate for children [50, 51]. Palpation for lymphadenopathy and organomegaly should also be performed, as they may suggest spread to regional lymph nodes or neighboring organs.

Valuable laboratory tests to obtain in the workup of MF include a complete blood count (CBC) with differential, comprehensive metabolic panel (CMP), lactate dehydrogenase level, absolute Sézary cell count using flow cytometry, and TCR gene rearrangement. In particular within the CBC, absolute lymphocyte counts should be assessed. Further, review of the peripheral blood smear for Sézary cells and liver enzymes for hepatic involvement should also be completed. Although lymph nodes are the most frequent location of extracutaneous MF, hepatic involvement has also been observed in the literature [52]. As mentioned previously, flow cytometry provides a helpful quantitative assessment of the abnormal T-lymphocyte phenotype. The flow cytometry is optional for patients in early phase Stage 1 disease, and is recommended for patients with stage 2 disease or greater, observed lymphadenopathy, or suspected extracutaneous manifestations. Similarly, TCR gene rearrangement studies in blood are recommended for patients with suspected blood involvement, given the high frequency of clonal TCR gene rearrangements at MF patients with advanced, systemic stages. Imaging studies, including computed tomography (CT) with contrast or PET/CT, may also be needed to confirm suspected visceral involvement, particularly for patients with advanced stage MF greater than T2.

Additional workup components may also be situationally employed when needed in certain circumstances. Dependent on the presentation, additional biopsies may be required. These include rebiopsy of skin lesions, biopsy of suspicious lymph nodes when lymphadenopathy is observed, biopsy of suspicious extracutaneous sites, and bone marrow biopsy. Bone marrow biopsies are generally only recommended following proven malignant blood or nodal infiltration. Finally, pregnancy testing or fertility discussions may need to be taken into account when considering treatment options that are contraindicated in pregnancy or that may impact fertility.

References

[1] Hodak, E. and I. Amitay-Laish, Mycosis fungoides: A great imitator. *Clin Dermatol*, 2019. 37(3): p. 255-267.

[2] Zackheim, H. S. and T. H. McCalmont, Mycosis fungoides: the great imitator. *J Am Acad Dermatol,* 2002. 47(6): p. 914-8.

[3] Cerroni, L., Mycosis fungoides-clinical and histopathologic features, differential diagnosis, and treatment. *Semin Cutan Med Surg*, 2018. 37(1): p. 2-10.

[4] Olsen, E. A., et al., Clinical end points and response criteria in mycosis fungoides and Sézary syndrome: a consensus statement of the International Society for Cutaneous Lymphomas, the United States Cutaneous Lymphoma Consortium, and the Cutaneous Lymphoma Task Force of the European Organisation for Research and Treatment of Cancer. *J Clin Oncol,* 2011. 29(18): p. 2598-607.

[5] Vaidya, T. and T. Badri, Mycosis Fungoides, in *StatPearls*. 2020: Treasure Island (FL).

[6] Huang, A. H., et al., Racial Disparities in the Clinical Presentation and Prognosis of Patients with Mycosis Fungoides. *J Natl Med Assoc*, 2019. 111(6): p. 633-639.

[7] Geller, S., et al., Understanding racial disparities in mycosis fungoides through international collaborative studies. *Br J Dermatol*, 2019. 180(5): p. 1263-1264.

[8] Alsayyah, A., Is it mycosis fungoides? A comprehensive guide to reaching the diagnosis and avoiding common pitfalls. *Annals of Diagnostic Pathology*, 2020. 47: p. 151546.

[9] Galper, S. L., B. D. Smith, and L. D. Wilson, Diagnosis and management of mycosis fungoides. *Oncology* (Williston Park, N.Y.), 2010. 24(6): p. 491-501.

[10] Sokołowska-Wojdyło, M., K. Olek-Hrab, and K. Ruckemann-Dziurdzińska, Primary cutaneous lymphomas: diagnosis and treatment. *Advances in Dermatology and Allergology/Postępy Dermatologii i Alergologii*, 2015. 32(5): p. 368-383.

[11] Sutton, A., et al., Selection of biopsy type and site for accurate diagnosis of mycosis fungoides: A single institution experience. *Journal of the American Academy of Dermatology*, 2017. 76(6): p. AB233.

[12] Elston, D. M., E. J. Stratman, and S. J. Miller, Skin biopsy: Biopsy issues in specific diseases. *Journal of the American Academy of Dermatology*, 2016. 74(1): p. 1-16.

[13] Agarwal, S. and K. Krishnamurthy, Histology, Skin, in *StatPearls*. 2020, StatPearls Publishing: Treasure Island (FL).

[14] Dewar, R., et al., Best Practices in Diagnostic Immunohistochemistry: Workup of Cutaneous Lymphoid Lesions in the Diagnosis of Primary Cutaneous Lymphoma. *Archives of Pathology & Laboratory Medicine*, 2015. 139(3): p. 338-350.

[15] Olek-Hrab, K. and W. Silny, Diagnostics in mycosis fungoides and Sézary syndrome. *Reports of Practical Oncology and Radiotherapy*, 2013. 19(2): p. 72-76.

[16] Harvey, N. T., D. V. Spagnolo, and B. A. Wood, 'Could it be mycosis fungoides?': an approach to diagnosing patch stage mycosis fungoides. *Journal of Hematopathology*, 2015. 8(4): p. 209-223.

[17] Pulitzer, M. P., P. Horna, and J. Almeida, Sézary syndrome and mycosis fungoides: An overview, including the role of immunophenotyping. *Cytometry Part B: Clinical Cytometry*, 2020. 100(2): p. 132-138.

[18] Murphy, M., D. Fullen, and J. A. Carlson, Low CD7 expression in benign and malignant cutaneous lymphocytic infiltrates: experience with an antibody reactive with paraffin-embedded tissue. *The American Journal of Dermatopathology*, 2002. 24(1): p. 6-16.

[19] Hodges, E., et al., Diagnostic role of tests for T cell receptor (TCR) genes. *Journal of Clinical Pathology*, 2003. 56(1): p. 1-11.

[20] Ponti, R., et al., T-cell receptor gamma gene rearrangement by multiplex polymerase chain reaction/heteroduplex analysis in patients with cutaneous T-cell lymphoma (mycosis fungoides/Sézary syndrome) and benign inflammatory disease: correlation with clinical,

histological and immunophenotypical findings. *The British Journal of Dermatology*, 2005. 153(3): p. 565-573.

[21] Rea, B., et al., Role of high-throughput sequencing in the diagnosis of cutaneous T-cell lymphoma. *Journal of Clinical Pathology*, 2018. 71(9): p. 814-820.

[22] Jokinen, C. H., et al., Flow Cytometric Evaluation of Skin Biopsies for Mycosis Fungoides. *The American Journal of Dermatopathology*, 2011. 33(5): p. 483-491.

[23] Amatore, F., et al., ICOS is widely expressed in cutaneous T-cell lymphoma, and its targeting promotes potent killing of malignant cells. *Blood Advances*, 2020. 4(20): p. 5203-5214.

[24] Lu, D., et al., The T-cell chemokine receptor CXCR3 is expressed highly in low-grade mycosis fungoides. *American Journal of Clinical Pathology*, 2001. 115(3): p. 413-421.

[25] Michie, S. A., et al., Expression of T-cell receptor antigens in mycosis fungoides and inflammatory skin lesions. *The Journal of Investigative Dermatology*, 1989. 93(1): p. 116-120.

[26] O'Malley, D. P., et al., Utility of BCL2, PD1, and CD25 immunohistochemical expression in the diagnosis of T-cell lymphomas. Applied immunohistochemistry & molecular morphology: *AIMM*, 2014. 22(2): p. 99-104.

[27] Vermeer, M. H., et al., Expression of cytotoxic proteins by neoplastic T cells in mycosis fungoides increases with progression from plaque stage to tumor stage disease. *The American Journal of Pathology*, 1999. 154(4): p. 1203-1210.

[28] Hristov, A. C., E. C. Vonderheid, and M. J. Borowitz, Simplified Flow Cytometric Assessment in Mycosis Fungoides and Sézary Syndrome. *American Journal of Clinical Pathology*, 2011. 136(6): p. 944-953.

[29] Netchiporouk, E., et al., Analysis of CTCL cell lines reveals important differences between mycosis fungoides/Sézary syndrome vs. HTLV-1 + leukemic cell lines. *Oncotarget,* 2017. 8(56): p. 95981-95998.

[30] Eusebio-Ponce, E., et al., HTLV-1 infection: An emerging risk. Pathogenesis, epidemiology, diagnosis and associated diseases. *Rev Esp Quimioter*, 2019. 32(6): p. 485-496.

[31] Hsi, A. C., et al., Expression of helper T cell master regulators in inflammatory dermatoses and primary cutaneous T-cell lymphomas: diagnostic implications. *Journal of the American Academy of Dermatology,* 2015. 72(1): p. 159-167.

[32] Schrader, A. M. R., P. M. Jansen, and R. Willemze, TOX expression in cutaneous T-cell lymphomas: an adjunctive diagnostic marker that is not tumour specific and not restricted to the CD4(+) CD8(-) phenotype. *The British Journal of Dermatology,* 2016. 175(2): p. 382-386.

[33] Dulmage, B., et al., The biomarker landscape in mycosis fungoides and Sézary syndrome. *Experimental Dermatology*, 2017. 26(8): p. 668-676.

[34] Hoppe, R. T., et al., CD8-positive tumor-infiltrating lymphocytes influence the long-term survival of patients with mycosis fungoides. *J Am Acad Dermatol*, 1995. 32(3): p. 448-53.

[35] Meissner, K., et al., Epidermal Langerhans' cell densities influence survival in mycosis fungoides and Sézary syndrome. *Cancer,* 1990. 65(9): p. 2069-73.

[36] Wu, X., et al., Depletion of M2-like tumor-associated macrophages delays cutaneous T-cell lymphoma development *in vivo. J Invest Dermatol*, 2014. 134(11): p. 2814-2822.

[37] Gjerdrum, L. M., et al., FOXP3+ regulatory T cells in cutaneous T-cell lymphomas: association with disease stage and survival. *Leukemia*, 2007. 21(12): p. 2512-8.

[38] Ni, X., et al., Reduction of regulatory T cells by Mogamulizumab, a defucosylated anti-CC chemokine receptor 4 antibody, in patients with aggressive/refractory mycosis fungoides and Sézary syndrome. *Clin Cancer Res*, 2015. 21(2): p. 274-85.

[39] Fernandes, I. C., et al., Can the level of CD52 expression on Sézary cells be used to predict the response of Sézary syndrome to

alemtuzumab? *Journal of the American Academy of Dermatology*, 2012. 67(5): p. 1083-1085.

[40] Kantekure, K., et al., Expression patterns of the immunosuppressive proteins PD-1/CD279 and PD-L1/CD274 at different stages of cutaneous T-cell lymphoma (CTCL)/mycosis fungoides (MF). *The American Journal of Dermatopathology*, 2012. 34(1): p. 126-128.

[41] Mehra, T., et al., Brentuximab as a Treatment for CD30 + Mycosis Fungoides and Sézary Syndrome. *JAMA Dermatology*, 2015. 151(1): p. 73.

[42] Moins-Teisserenc, H., et al., CD158k is a reliable marker for diagnosis of Sézary syndrome and reveals an unprecedented heterogeneity of circulating malignant cells. *The Journal of Investigative Dermatology*, 2015. 135(1): p. 247-257.

[43] Prince, H. M., et al., Denileukin diftitox for the treatment of CD25 low-expression mycosis fungoides and Sézary syndrome. *Leukemia & Lymphoma*, 2013. 54(1): p. 69-75.

[44] Sugaya, M., et al., CCR4 is expressed on infiltrating cells in lesional skin of early mycosis fungoides and atopic dermatitis. *The Journal of Dermatology*, 2015. 42(6): p. 613-615.

[45] Jankowska-Konsur, A., et al., Expression of SATB1, MTI/II and Ki-67 in Mycosis Fungoides. *Anticancer Research,* 2016. 36(1): p. 189-197.

[46] Goswami, M., et al., Increased Twist expression in advanced stage of Mycosis fungoides and Sézary syndrome. *Journal of cutaneous pathology*, 2012. 39(5): p. 500-507.

[47] Raghavan, S. S., et al., Utility of CD30, Ki-67, and p53 in assisting with the diagnosis of mycosis fungoides with large cell transformation. *Journal of Cutaneous Pathology,* 2018. 46(1): p. 33-43.

[48] Nielsen, S., External quality assessment for immunohistochemistry: experiences from NordiQC. *Biotechnic & Histochemistry: Official Publication of the Biological Stain Commission*, 2015. 90(5): p. 331-340.

[49] Anagnostou, V. K., et al., Analytic Variability in Immunohistochemistry Biomarker Studies. Cancer epidemiology,

biomarkers & prevention: a *publication of the American Association for Cancer Research,* cosponsored by the American Society of Preventive Oncology, 2010. 19(4): p. 982-991.

[50] Rhodes, J., C. Clay, and M. Phillips, The surface area of the hand and the palm for estimating percentage of total body surface area: results of a meta-analysis. *The British Journal of Dermatology,* 2013. 169(1): p. 76-84.

[51] Scarisbrick, J. J. and S. Morris, How big is your hand and should you use it to score skin in cutaneous T-cell lymphoma? *The British Journal of Dermatology*, 2013. 169(2): p. 260-265.

[52] Malik, N. and I. Weisberg, Mycosis Fungoides of the Liver: 2267. *Official journal of the American College of Gastroenterology* 2017. 112: p. S1244.

In: Mycosis Fungoides and Sézary Syndrome ISBN: 978-1-68507-093-9
Editors: X. Zhang and L. Sokol

Chapter 3

PATHOLOGICAL FEATURES AND DIAGNOSIS OF MYCOSIS FUNGOIDES

Xiaohui Zhang**, MD, PhD
Department of Pathology,
H. Lee Moffitt Cancer Center and Research Institute, Tampa, FL, USA

INTRODUCTION

Mycosis fungoides (MF) is the most common subtype of cutaneous lymphoma with distinct clinical and pathological features. Clinically, it is initially an indolent disease with a primary presentation on skin, which is usually scaly, well-demarcated skin plaques and patches that are refractory to treatment, and in the later stages, it can progress to tumors and erythroderma, and can ultimately develop lymphadenopathy and/or hepatosplenomegaly. Histopathologically, MF is characterized by epidermal and dermal infiltrates of small to medium-sized atypical lymphoid cells with cerebriform nuclei. It can be very challenging to diagnose MF, particularly

* Corresponding Author's Email: xiaohui.zhang@moffitt.org.

at early stages, since it can mimic and overlap with benign dermatoses and other T cell lymphomas, both clinically and pathologically. In addition, there are many clinical and histologic variants of MF, further complicating the clinical and pathological diagnoses. In this chapter, we will address the histologic features of MF, diagnostic algorithm, features of MF pathological variants recognized by WHO-EORTC classification, and the major differential diagnoses for MF.

Histologic Features and Diagnosis

The histological hallmark of MF is epidermotropism, which is the infiltration of epidermis by small to medium sized atypical lymphocytes with enlarged hyperchromatic, cerebriform nuclei and clear cytoplasm (haloed cells) (Fig. 3-1). These atypical lymphocytes can be singly scattered or form a linear distribution along the basal layer of the epidermis ("string of pearls") (Fig. 3-1). Approximately 25% of MF can have small aggregates of atypical lymphocytes within the epidermis, often in association with Langerhans cells, which are called "Pautrier microabscesses" (Fig. 3-2) and are considered to be a typical histological feature of MF [1], although it is not unique in MF and can be seen in other cutaneous T cell processes such as adult T-cell leukemia/lymphoma (ATLL), actinic reticuloid and drug-induced T-cell pseudolymphomas. Epidermotropism differs from exocytosis of lymphocytes, which is a term often used to describe benign conditions such as dermatitis and eczema, in which there is cytologic atypia with no or only very mild spongiosis (spaces between neighboring keratinocytes are enlarged by intense edema). Exocytosis often shows a pagetoid distribution pattern of lymphocytes, in contrast to basilar/lentiginous pattern seen in MF [2].

In early patch lesions, epidermis usually shows normal thickness, can be slightly acanthotic or atrophic, and may have mild hyperkeratosis with focal parakeratosis. Basal cell vacuolar degeneration can occur, in which the cells in the dermo-epidermal junctions become vacuolated and ill-defined as a result of basal cell degeneration. Within the epidermis, there are small numbers of atypical lymphocytes, in which clear halos may not be evident, and occasionally, few larger atypical cells may also be seen. In superficial dermis, band-like or lichenoid lymphocyte infiltrates are present. It can be perivascular lymphohistiocytic infiltrate surrounding superficial vascular plexus and extending into the papillary dermis [3] (Fig. 3-3).

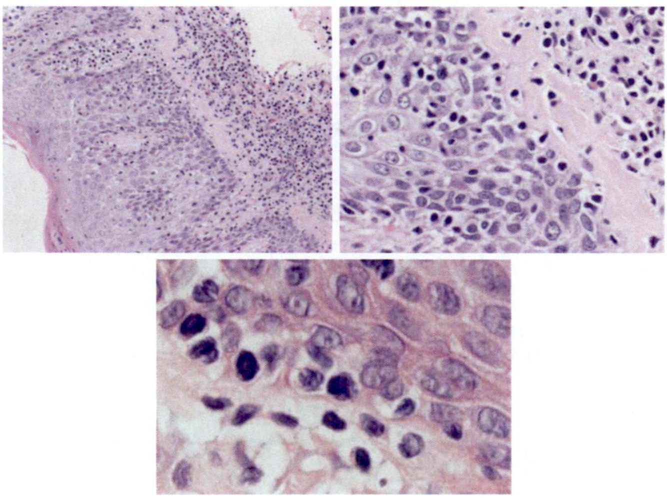

Figure 3-1. Epidermotropism in mycosis fungoides (patch stage). A. Atypical lymphocytes with hyperchromatic, cerebreform nuclei and clear cytoplasm infiltrate into epidermis. B and C. The atypical lymphocytes form a linear distribution along the dermoepidermal junction ("string of pearls") (C, courtesy of Dr. Haipeng Shao, H. Lee Moffitt Cancer Center).

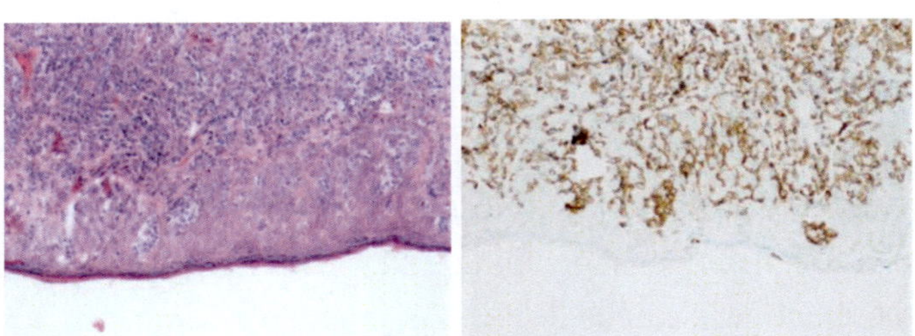

Figure 3-2. Pautrier microabscesses formation in mycosis fungoides. A. Small aggregates of atypical lymphocytes form within the epidermis ("Pautrier microabscesses"). B. CD3 immunostain.

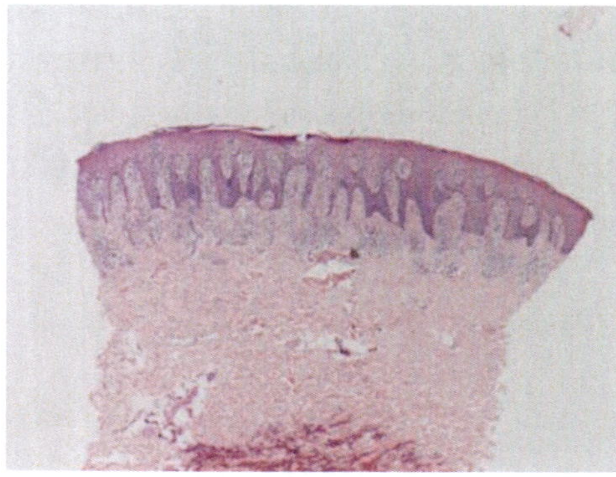

Figure 3-3. Band-like atypical lymphocyte infiltrate in the superficial dermis. Epidermotropism is present in this patch stage of mycosis fungoides.

In typical plaque stage MF, epidermis is commonly acanthotic, and can have compact hyperkeratosis and patchy parakeratosis, resembling a psoriasiform appearance. Epidermotropism is more pronounced and superficial dermal band-like atypical lymphocytic infiltrate is more intense. Pautrier microabscesses can be seen in some cases [4]. Reactive inflammatory cells, including eosinophils, plasma cells, and histiocytes, can be present.

In tumor stage MF, the dermal infiltrates are intense, sometimes extending into the subcutaneous fat. However, the epidermotropism may be subtle or absent. The infiltrate may be diffuse or shows a vaguely nodular pattern, and oftentimes, the neoplastic lymphocytes are more pleomorphic, showing variable proportions of small, medium-sized lymphocytes, large cerebriform cells, blastic cells with prominent nuclei and intermediate forms [5]. Mitotic figures are frequent and pathologic mitosis may be seen.

Immunophenotypically, in large majority of MF cases, the neoplastic lymphocytes are CD4+ T cells expressing T cell receptor (TCR) β (βF1) and variable pan-T cell antigens including CD2, CD3, CD5 and CD7 [6]. One or more of these antigens can be lost. CD7 is the most commonly lost marker, followed by CD5, CD2 and even CD3. CD7 loss can occur in all stages of MF [6], particularly patch stage MF (Fig. 3-4), while aberrant expression of CD5, CD2 and CD3 usuallly is the finding in late stages (plaque and tumor stages) of MF. It is noteworthy to mention that it is helpful to assess epidermal component and dermal component independently, since dermal component may contain numerous reactive lymphocytes that can obscure the antigen loss in neoplastic T cells [1]. CD7 immunostain is helpful in the MF diagnosis [7]. However, practically, CD7 antigen immunostain is most reliable in frozen sections, and diminished staining is observed in tissue sections fixed with formalin for longer than 24 hours [8], which warrants careful evaluation of CD7 stain in the diagnosis of difficult MF cases, particularly for those with prolonged fixation [9].

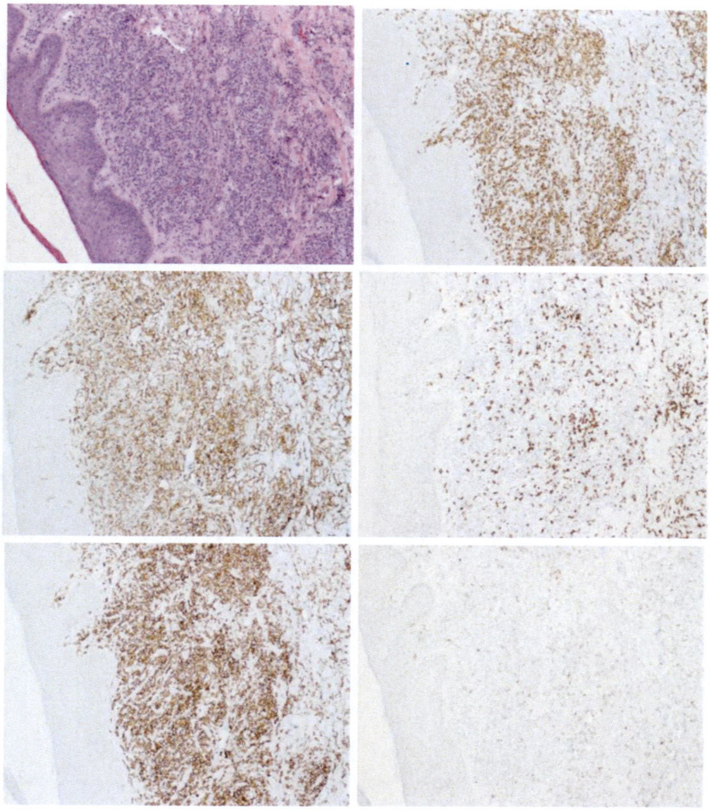

Figure 3-4. CD7 loss is the most frequent aberrancy seen in mycosis fungoides. A. Dense atypical lymphocytic infiltrate is present in this tumor stage of mycosis fungoides. There is only minimal epidermotropism in this case. B-F. Immunostains show that the neoplastic T cells are CD3+ (B), CD4+ (C), CD8- (D), CD5+ (E), and CD7- (F).

A subset of MF cases can show a CD8+ phenotype [10] (Fig. 3-5), which is more commonly found in pediatric MF [11] and associated with hypo- and hyper-pigmented lesions [12, 13]. CD8+ cases may have a cytotoxic immunophenotype. CD8+ MF does not behave differently than CD4+ MF [14]. Rarer cases can even show CD56+ phenotype, which may be CD4 or CD8 positive [15]. CD30 is mainly expressed in tumor stage, particularly in transformed cells, although its expression can be detected in plaque stage [16].

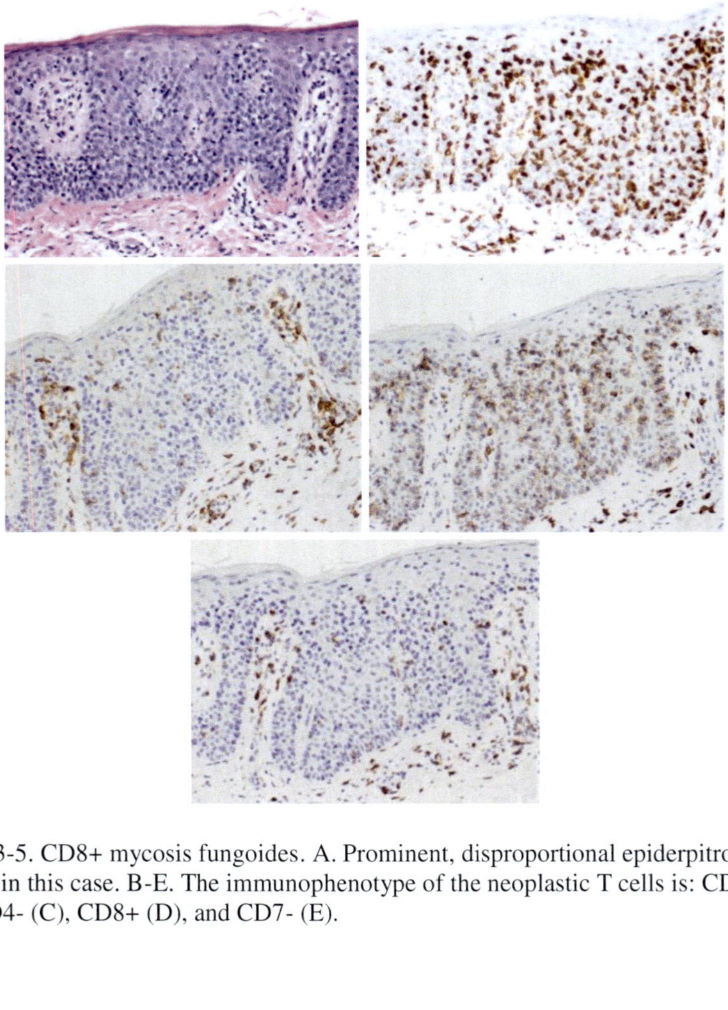

Figure 3-5. CD8+ mycosis fungoides. A. Prominent, disproportional epiderpitropism is present in this case. B-E. The immunophenotype of the neoplastic T cells is: CD3+ (B), CD4- (C), CD8+ (D), and CD7- (E).

Clonal TCR beta and/or gamma gene rearrangement can be identified by polymerase chain reaction (PCR)-based testing in the majority of cases. However, benign inflammatory dermatoses can show clonal TCR gene rearrangement too [17, 18], and false negative results can be resulted possibly due to scarcity of the cells in early MF cases. Therefore, when interpreting TCR gene rearrangement results, extreme caution needs to be taken and it cannot be used as the sole criterion to establish a diagnosis of MF. The results can be used in conjunction with clinical presentation and histologic findings.

Flow cytometry has been reported to be a useful tool in identifying neoplastic T cell populations in skin biopsies [19-21]. Although it shows certain advantages over immunohistochemistry including separating the aberrant lymphoid subsets from normal lymphocytes by simultaneously evaluating multiple T cell antigens, the unilization of the method in diagnosis of MF, particularly early stage MF, is limited by paucicellularity and lack of analysis of sensitivity and specificity [20].

There is an emerging utilization of TCR constant β chain-1 (TRBC1) marker by flow cytometric analysis in the diagnosis of MF [22]. The marker is specific for one of two mutually exclusive TRBC1 expression and can be used to determine the clonality of the T-cells. This simple and rapid assay could be routinely utilized in the flow cytometry laboratories [23, 24].

It can be challenging to make a definitive diagnosis of a patch or early plaque stage MF with subtle changes, in which ancillary studies including immunophenotyping, TCR gene rearrangement analysis by PCR, may be helpful in aiding the diagnosis. Correlation with clinical presentation is very important, although clinical information and pathologic features can be conflicting. To improve the accuracy of diagnosis, an algorithm for diagnosing early MF is developed in 2005 by the International Society for Cutaneous Lymphoma (ISCL) based on the combined approach of using both clinical and pathological criteria (Table 3-1) [25].

Table 3-1. Algorithm for diagnosis of early stage mycosis mungoides

Criteria	**Scoring System (Points) by Criteria**
1. Clinical	2 (basic plus 2 additional); 1 (basic plus 1 additional)
Basic Persistent and/or progressive patches/thin plaques Additional 1) Non–sun-exposed location 2) Size/shape variation 3) Poikiloderma	
2. Histopathologic	2 (basic plus 2 additional); 1 (basic plus 1 additional)
Basic Superficial lymphoid infiltrate Additional 1) Epidermotropism without spongiosis 2) Lymphoid atypia	
3. Molecular (clonality)	1 (clonality)
Clonal T-cell receptor gene rearrangement	
4. Immunophenotypic (1 or more criteria)	1 (1 or more criteria)
1) <50% CD2+, CD3+, and/or CD5+ T cells 2) <10% CD7+ T cells 3) T-cell antigen loss confined to epidermis	

Adapted and modified from Pimpinelli et al., [25].

* A total of 4 points is required for the diagnosis of MF based on any combination of points from the clinical, histopathologic, molecular, and immunophenotypic criteria.

MF Variants

Besides classical MF, there are many clinical and histologic variants of MF. Three distinct variants, folliculotropic MF, pagetoid reticulosis, and granulomatous slack skin, show distinctive clinicopathologic features, and have been recognized in WHO-EORTC classification [5]. Additionally, different clinical variants such as bullous and hyper- or hypopigmented MF, and histological variants such as granulomatous MF and syringotropic MF have been described [26].

Folliculotropic MF

Folliculotropic MF, used to be called follicular mucinosis, is characterized by the presence of folliculotropic CD4+ neoplastic T cell infiltrates (folliculotropism), often with sparing of the epidermis, and with frequent concomitant follicular mucinosis, which is mucinous degeneration of the hair follicles. Cases without follicular mucinosis have been called as folliculocentric or pilotropic MF, and show no differences in clinical presentation and clinical behavior from cases with associated follicular mucinosis [27, 28]. Folliculotropic MF commonly involves the head and neck and is often associated with alopecia and occasionally mucinorrhea. Clinically the patients may present as patches, erythematous indurated plaques, grouped papules or tumors.

Histologic findings of folliculotropic MF include the primarily perivascular and periadnexal localization of the dermal infiltrates with variable infiltration of the follicutropic small, medium-sized, or sometimes large hyperchromatic neoplastic T cells with cerebriform nuclei (Fig. 3-6). Follicular mucinosis can be assessed with Alcian blue staining. Admixed eosinophils and plasma cells can be seen. It should be noted that mucin within follicles can occur in other clinical settings such as alopecia mucinosa, thus is not specific for folliculotropic MF [29].

Folliculotropic MF is more difficult to treat than classic MF, and has a higher incidence of disease progression with worse prognosis [30, 31]. This is possibly due to the perifollicular localization of the dermal infiltrates which is more refractory to skin-targeted treatment such as PUVA and topical nitrogen mustard. The treatment opitons include total skin electron beam irradiation, PUVA combined with retinoids or interferon alpha, and local radiotherapy to persistent tumors [5, 31].

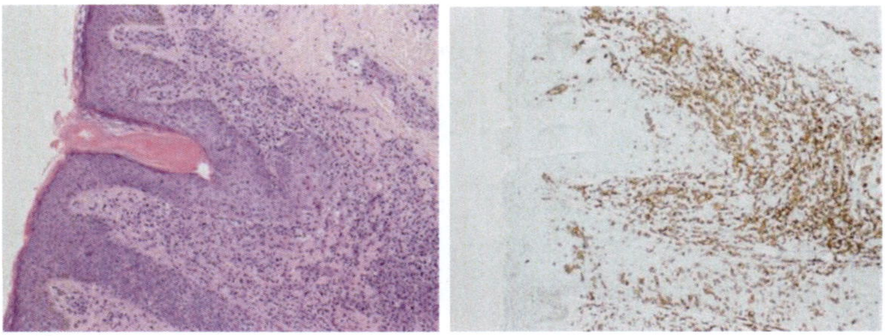

Figure 3-6. A. Follicutropic small to medium-sized hyperchromatic neoplastic T cells in folliculotropic mycosis fungoides. B. CD3 immunostain.

Pagetoid Reticulosis

Pagetoid reticulosis is a variant of MF characterized by the presence of localized patches or plaques with a disproportionate intraepidermal proliferation of neoplastic T cells [32]. This entity was initially described by Woringer and Kolopp in two children, and the term pagetoid reticulosis should only be used for the localized type (Woringer-Kolopp type) and not for the disseminated type (Ketron-Goodman type) [33], which would likely be classified as aggressive epidermotropic CD8+ CTCL, cutaneous gamma/delta-positive T-cell lymphoma, or tumor stage MF [5].

The affected skin in pagetoid reticulosis is usually on the extremities. Clinical presentations are warty, hyperkeratotic plaques on the hands and feet. The histologic features include a hyperplastic epidermis with marked infiltration by atypical pagetoid cells which are medium or large sized with hyperchromatic and cerebriform nuclei, singly or arranged in nests. In the dermis, there may be benign lymphohistiocytic infiltrate, but no neoplastic T cells [32]. Immunophenotypically, the neoplastic T cells may be either CD4+ or CD8+. CD30 is often expressed [34] (Fig. 3-7).

The prognosis of pagetoid reticulosis is far better than that of classic MF. Many patients can achieve remission by localized therapies, such as excision or radiation. Extracutaneous dissemination or disease-related deaths have never been reported [5].

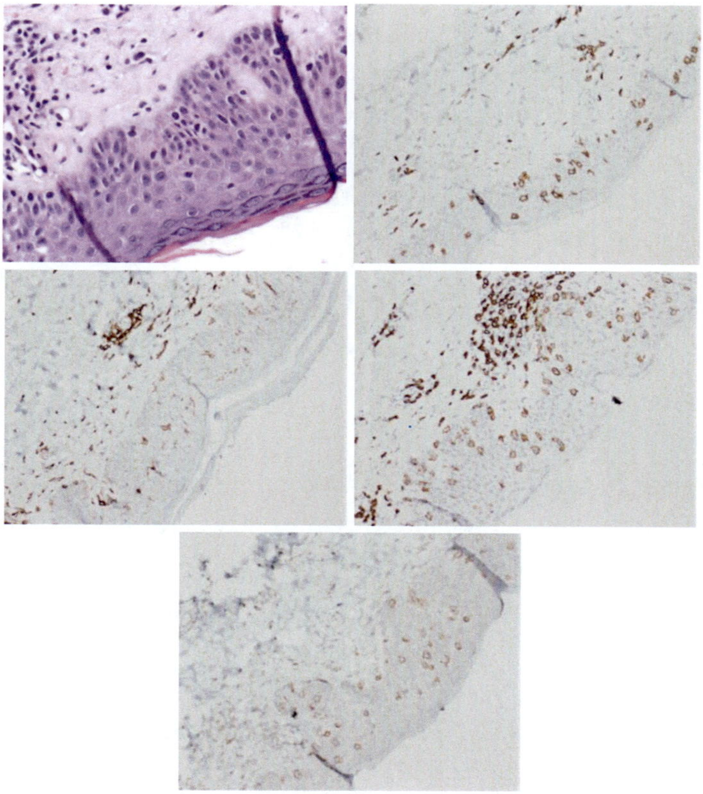

Figure 3-7. Pagetoid reticulosis. A. Intraepidermal pegetoid distribution of the atypical lymphocytes with hyperchromatic and cerebreform nuclei. B-E. Characteristic immunophenotype of the neoplastic T cells: CD3+ (B), CD4- (C), CD8+ (D), and CD30+ (E).

Granulomatous Slack Skin

Granulomatous slack skin (GSS) is an extremely uncommon MF variant characterized by the development of erythematous loose skin masses in major skin folds and histologically by a granulomatous infiltrate with clonal T cells [35]. The patients present with pendulous lax skin, or bulky skin folds, with a predilection for the axillae and groins. Histologically, there are diffuse infiltrates of atypical lymphocytes extending throughout the entire dermis and the subcutis, dense granulomatous changes with many macrophages and often multinucleated giant cells, and destruction of elastic tissue. Epidermotropism is not a prominent feature but may be focally present [36]. The atypical lymphocytes show CD3+, CD4+, CD8- phenotype. Monoclonal TCR gene rearrangements have been identified in almost all cases. In one-third of the cases association with Hodgkin lymphoma was observed [5, 35, 37-39]. Clinical course is usually indolent and the progression is slow over years.

Other Histologic Variants

Rare cases show unusual histological features with undetermined clinical significance. Though currently they are not recognized as biologically distinct variants, they have been designated with different specific names and the histological patterns have been well illustrated.

Syringotropic MF

Syringotropic MF is a rare variant of MF characterized by a particular tropism of the lymphocytic infiltrate for the eccrine structures, and has been included in the follicular MF in the WHO–EORTC classification [5]. As a matter of fact, a subset of follicular MF cases can have prominent infiltration of both follicular epithelium and eccrine sweat glands. The syringotropic MF skin lesions are usually localized, with erythematous or brown patches and plaques with superimposed papules, often accompanied by hair loss [40]. Histologically, there are dense atypical lymphocyte infiltrates surrounding eccrine secretory coils in addition to infiltrates elsewhere in the dermis and epidermis [41, 42]. Although clinical behavior of this rare variant is not completely clear, there was a report that syringotropic MF had more favorable prognosis than follicular MF [43].

Granulomatous MF

Granulomatous MF is another rare variant of MF characterized by an infiltrate of atypical lymphocytes, with histiocyte proliferation ranging from loose clusters of histiocytes and scattered multinucleated giant cells to well-formed granulomas [36]. Granulomatous MF and granulomatous slack skin share similar histologic features and only differ by clinical presentation. Clinically, granulomatous MF is indistinguishable from typical MF, with presentation of papule, plaque or tumor. Granulomas are thought to be an inflammatory reaction change. Special stains for microorganisms should be performed to exclude an infection. Contrary to the initial report that granulomatous MF had favorable outcome, more recent studies have shown that extracutaneous manifestations are more frequent in granulomatous MF and occur earlier than in classical MF, and five year survival rate of granulomatous MF is worse than that of classical MF [44].

Clinical Variants

MF patients may have unusual clinical presentations with similar clinical course and outcome to typical MF. There are a wide range of rare atypical presentations described in the literature, including hypopigmented, hyperpigmented, verrucous, hyperkeratotic, lichenoid papular, palmoplantar psoriasiform, vesicular, bullous, and pustular variants [45]. Below are few examples.

Poikilodermatous MF

This variant was described in 1906 by the American pediatrician Abraham Jacobi as a complex dermatologic disease characterized by telangiectasia, hyper- and hypo-pigmentation, and atrophy, which he subsequently termed poikiloderma vasculare atrophicans (PVA) [46, 47]. Histopathologically poikilodermatous MF shows atypical T cell infiltrate in the papillary dermis with epidermotropism, epidermal atrophy, dilated blood vessels in the dermis, melanophages, and melanin incontinence [48]. Poikilodermatous MF has similar prognosis to typical MF [49].

Hypopigmented MF and Hyperpigmented MF

MF associated with either hypopigmentation or hyperpigmentation is rare. Hypopigmented MF occurs early in life and is seen in children and adolescents [50, 51]. Some author suggested that the presence of hypopigmentation may be considered as a marker of good prognosis [52]. Histologically, hypopigmented MF is usually indistinguishable from typical MF except for the presence of pigment incontinence. Rare cases manifest as hyperpigmentated lesions [53], and the phenotype is predominantly CD8+ [13].

Bullous MF

Bullous MF is extremely rare and is characterized by localized or generalized blisters, which can occur on normal skin, or within the patches, plaques and tumors of MF [54]. Histologically, the atypical lymphocytes replace basal keratinocytes, resulting in clefts between the epidermis and dermis [55].

Differential Diagnosis

Many benign skin diseases such as reactive inflammatory conditions can share similar histological and even clinical features with MF, particularly the patch stage. These include nonspecific dermatitis, spongiotic dermatitis, interface dermatitides, contact dermatitis, drug eruption, and other conditions (also see Chapter 5. *Differential diagnosis of early mycosis fungoides and benign dermatoses*). Other cutaneous T cell lymphomas can also mimick MF/SS.

Nonspecific Dermatitis

The histologic findings that may be helpful in distinguising MF from nonspecific dermatitis are listed in Table 3-2 [4, 56, 57].

Table 3-2. Useful histologic features in distinguishing MF from nonspecific dermatitis

Category	Histologic features	Comment
Cell atypia	1. Lymphocytes with convoluted nuclei, particularly in epidermis 2. Lymphocytes with surrounding halos 3. Epidermal lymphocytes larger than dermal lymphocytes.	Convoluted nuclei are very specific to MF. However, lymphocyte atypia is often not apparent in early lesions.
Cell arrangement	1. Lymphocytes arrange in linear array at the dermoepidermal junction 2. Pautrier microabscesses.	
Cell distribution	Disproportionate epidermotropism	
Other features	1. Eccrine infiltration 2. Follicular tropism 3. Follicular mucin 4. Absence of edema 5. Wiry bundles of papillary dermal collagen associated with a lichenoid infiltrate.	It has been reported that eccrine infiltration and follicular mucin are relatively specific findings to MF.

Spongiotic Dermatitis

In spongiotic dermatitis, the lymphocytic infiltrate is usually perivascular in the superficial dermis, comparing to band like infiltrate in MF. There is usually abundant spongiosis without many lymphocytes. Many spongiotic dermatitis cases have eosinophils in both the dermis and the epidermis, while early MF seldomly has more than a few eosinophils.

Interface Dermatitis

This is a group of diseases charaterized by prominent lymphocytic infiltrates obscuring the dermo-epidermal junction, including lichen planus, pityriasis lichenoides et varioliformis acuta (PLEVA), pityriasis lichenoides chronica (PLC), fixed durg eruption, lichen aureus, cutaneous lupus, toxic epidermal necrosis (Stevens-Johnson syndrome), and lymphomatoid drug reaction. The histologic changes can include damaged keratinocytes (forming Civatte bodies in epidermis and colloid bodies in papillary dermis), vacuolar change that is most prominent at the basal cell layer, and alteration of rete ridges that become serrated or recede entirely. The interface pattern can be seen in MF as small focal changes, but rarely become the dominant features.

Drug Eruption

Drug eruptions can simulate early stage MF. MF-like skin reactions to antiepileptic drugs such as phenytoin, carbamazepine, oxcarbazepine, phenobarbital have been reported [58, 59]. The clinical history is the key to making the diagnosis, and the lesion should be resolved after the insulting medication is suspended.

Lymphomatoid Allergic Contact Dermatitis

This unusual type of allergic contact dermatitis can show superficial and deep perivascular lymphocytic infiltrate with variable degrees of spongiosis, epidermotropism, and cytological atypia, mimicking MF [60, 61]. If present, epidermal spongiosis or spongiotic microvesiculation may favor lymphomatoid contact dermatitis over MF. Accurate diagnosis depends on consideration of the clinical history, and pathological, immunohistochemical and molecular data [61].

Other Cutaneous or Systemic T Cell Lymphomas

Other types of cutaneous T cell lymphomas, like lymphomatoid papulosis, skin involvement by peripheral T cell lymphoma, skin involvement by adult T cell leukemia (HTLV-1+), primary aggressive CD8+ epidermotropic T cell lymphoma, and primary cutaneous gamma-delta T cell lymphoma, need to be differentiated from MF. In particular, type B lymphomatoid papulosis is very difficult to be distinguished from MF histologically, and the difference is mainly clinical. Lymphomatoid papulosis lesions can regress spontaneously. MF with large cell transformation needs to be differentiated from primary cutaneous anaplastic large cell lymphoma. Most MF with large cell transformation cases do not have >75% anaplastic CD30+ large cells, and show more heterogeneous cytology when comparing with primary cutaneous anaplastic large cell lymphoma. Still, it needs to be kept in mind that tumor stage MF can have sheets of anaplastic large lymphoid cells with diffuse expression of CD30, which has much worse prognosis than primary cutaneous anaplastic large cell lymphoma. Tumor stage MF may also be impossible to distinguish from skin involvement by peripheral T cell lymphoma, not otherwise specified, although the peripheral T cell lymphoma infiltrates are predominantly dermal. Only clinical presentation may tell these conditions apart. Histologically, it may also be problematic to differentiate other cutaneous T cell lymphomas from MF. Please also refer to Chapter 4 (*Pathological features of mycosis fungoides with large cell transformation*) for the differential diagnosis from other T cell lymphomas.

Conclusion

Histopathologically, MF has distinct architectural characteristics including epidermotropism, Pautrier microabscess formation, and marked lymphoid cell atypia. The histology varies in different stages of the disease. Immunophenotyping and flow cytometry can assist in the diagnosis. For the diagnosis of early MF, diagnostic algorithm has been developed, with criteria integrated the clinical, histopathologic, molecular and immunophenotypic findings. WHO-EORTC recognized MF variants include folliculotropic MF, pagetoid reticulosis and granulomatous slack skin, and other rarer clinical and histologic variants exist. The differential diagnosis can be difficult due to its overlap features with benign dermatoses and other primary cutaneous lymphomas.

REFERENCES

[1] Song, S. X., et al., Mycosis fungoides: report of the 2011 Society for Hematopathology/European Association for Haematopathology workshop. *Am J Clin Pathol*, 2013. 139(4): p. 466-90.

[2] Fung, M. A., 'Epidermotropism' vs. 'exocytosis' of lymphocytes 101: definition of terms. *J Cutan Pathol*, 2010. 37(5): p. 525-9.

[3] Massone, C., et al., Histopathologic features of early (patch) lesions of mycosis fungoides: a morphologic study on 745 biopsy specimens from 427 patients. *Am J Surg Pathol*, 2005. 29(4): p. 550-60.

[4] Smoller, B. R., et al., Reassessment of histologic parameters in the diagnosis of mycosis fungoides. *Am J Surg Pathol*, 1995. 19(12): p. 1423-30.

[5] Willemze, R., et al., WHO-EORTC classification for cutaneous lymphomas. *Blood*, 2005. 105(10): p. 3768-85.

[6] Ralfkiaer, E., Immunohistological markers for the diagnosis of cutaneous lymphomas. *Semin Diagn Pathol*, 1991. 8(2): p. 62-72.

[7] Cotta, A. C., et al., Diagnosis of mycosis fungoides: a comparative immunohistochemical study of T-cell markers using a novel anti-CD7 antibody. *Appl Immunohistochem Mol Morphol*, 2006. 14(3): p. 291-5.

[8] Murphy, M., D. Fullen, and J. A. Carlson, Low CD7 expression in benign and malignant cutaneous lymphocytic infiltrates: experience with an antibody reactive with paraffin-embedded tissue. *Am J Dermatopathol*, 2002. 24(1): p. 6-16.

[9] LeBoit, P. and L. Pincus, Mycosis fungoides and Sézary syndrome. in *Hematopathology*, E. Jaffe, et al., Editors. 2016, Elsevier: Philadelphia, PA. p. 713-729.

[10] Massone, C., et al., The prognosis of early mycosis fungoides is not influenced by phenotype and T-cell clonality. *Br J Dermatol,* 2008. 159(4): p. 881-6.

[11] Crowley, J. J., et al., Mycosis fungoides in young patients: clinical characteristics and outcome. *J Am Acad Dermatol*, 1998. 38(5 Pt 1): p. 696-701.

[12] El-Shabrawi-Caelen, L., et al., Hypopigmented mycosis fungoides: frequent expression of a CD8+ T-cell phenotype. *Am J Surg Pathol*, 2002. 26(4): p. 450-7.

[13] Pavlovsky, L., et al., Hyperpigmented mycosis fungoides: an unusual variant of cutaneous T-cell lymphoma with a frequent CD8+ phenotype. *J Am Acad Dermatol*, 2012. 67(1): p. 69-75.

[14] Diwan, H. and D. Ivan, CD8-positive mycosis fungoides and primary cutaneous aggressive epidermotropic CD8-positive cytotoxic T-cell lymphoma. *J Cutan Pathol*, 2009. 36(3): p. 390-2.

[15] Horst, B. A., R. Kasper, and P. E. LeBoit, CD4+, CD56+ mycosis fungoides: case report and review of the literature. *Am J Dermatopathol*, 2009. 31(1): p. 74-6.

[16] Wu, H., et al., Mycosis fungoides with CD30-positive cells in the epidermis. *Am J Dermatopathol*, 2000. 22(3): p. 212-6.

[17] Plaza, J. A., C. Morrison, and C. M. Magro, Assessment of TCR-beta clonality in a diverse group of cutaneous T-Cell infiltrates. *J Cutan Pathol*, 2008. 35(4): p. 358-65.

[18] Wood, G. S., et al., Detection of clonal T-cell receptor gamma gene rearrangements in early mycosis fungoides/Sézary syndrome by polymerase chain reaction and denaturing gradient gel electrophoresis (PCR/DGGE). *J Invest Dermatol*, 1994. 103(1): p. 34-41.

[19] Jokinen, C. H., et al., Flow cytometric evaluation of skin biopsies for mycosis fungoides. *Am J Dermatopathol*, 2011. 33(5): p. 483-91.

[20] Horna, P., et al., Flow cytometric identification of immunophenotypically aberrant T-cell clusters on skin shave biopsy

specimens from patients with mycosis fungoides. *Am J Clin Pathol*, 2015. 143(6): p. 785-96.

[21] Meyerson, H. J., Flow cytometry for the diagnosis of mycosis fungoides. *G Ital Dermatol Venereol*, 2008. 143(1): p. 21-41.

[22] Horna, P., et al., Emerging Role of T-cell Receptor Constant beta Chain-1 (TRBC1) Expression in the Flow Cytometric Diagnosis of T-cell Malignancies. *Int J Mol Sci*, 2021. 22(4).

[23] Shi, M., et al., Single Antibody Detection of T-Cell Receptor alphabeta Clonality by Flow Cytometry Rapidly Identifies Mature T-Cell Neoplasms and Monotypic Small CD8-Positive Subsets of Uncertain Significance. *Cytometry B Clin Cytom*, 2020. 98(1): p. 99-107.

[24] Berg, H., et al., Flow cytometric evaluation of TRBC1 expression in tissue specimens and body fluids is a novel and specific method for assessment of T-cell clonality and diagnosis of T-cell neoplasms. *Cytometry B Clin Cytom*, 2021. 100(3): p. 361-369.

[25] Pimpinelli, N., et al., Defining early mycosis fungoides. *J Am Acad Dermatol*, 2005. 53(6): p. 1053-63.

[26] Ahn, C. S., A. L. A, and O. P. Sangueza, Mycosis fungoides: an updated review of clinicopathologic variants. *Am J Dermatopathol*, 2014. 36(12): p. 933-48; quiz 949-51.

[27] Vergier, B., et al., Pilotropic cutaneous T-cell lymphoma without mucinosis. A variant of mycosis fungoides? French Study Group of Cutaneous Lymphomas. *Arch Dermatol*, 1996. 132(6): p. 683-7.

[28] Scheffer, C. J. and W. Back, Effects of 'navicular' shoeing on equine distal forelimb kinematics on different track surface. *Vet Q,* 2001. 23(4): p. 191-5.

[29] Cerroni, L., et al., Follicular mucinosis: a critical reappraisal of clinicopathologic features and association with mycosis fungoides and Sézary syndrome. *Arch Dermatol*, 2002. 138(2): p. 182-9.

[30] van Doorn, R., E. Scheffer, and R. Willemze, Follicular mycosis fungoides, a distinct disease entity with or without associated follicular mucinosis: a clinicopathologic and follow-up study of 51 patients. *Arch Dermatol*, 2002. 138(2): p. 191-8.

[31] Gerami, P., et al., Folliculotropic mycosis fungoides: an aggressive variant of cutaneous T-cell lymphoma. *Arch Dermatol*, 2008. 144(6): p. 738-46.

[32] Haghighi, B., et al., Pagetoid reticulosis (Woringer-Kolopp disease): an immunophenotypic, molecular, and clinicopathologic study. *Mod Pathol*, 2000. 13(5): p. 502-10.

[33] Swerdlow, S. H., International Agency for Research on Cancer and World Health Organization., WHO classification of tumours of haematopoietic and lymphoid tissues. 4th ed. *World Health Organization classification of tumours*. 2008, Lyon, France: International Agency for Research on Cancer.

[34] Jacyk, W. K., et al., Pagetoid reticulosis with CD30 positivity and cytotoxic/suppressor cells. *J Cutan Pathol*, 2007. 34(8): p. 644-7.

[35] van Haselen, C. W., et al., Granulomatous slack skin. Report of three patients with an updated review of the literature. *Dermatology*, 1998. 196(4): p. 382-91.

[36] Kempf, W., et al., Granulomatous mycosis fungoides and granulomatous slack skin: a multicenter study of the Cutaneous Lymphoma Histopathology Task Force Group of the European Organization for Research and Treatment of Cancer (EORTC). *Arch Dermatol*, 2008. 144(12): p. 1609-17.

[37] LeBoit, P. E., Granulomatous slack skin. *Dermatol Clin*, 1994. 12(2): p. 375-89.

[38] Clarijs, M., et al., Granulomatous slack skin: treatment with extensive surgery and review of the literature. *Dermatology*, 2003. 206(4): p. 393-7.

[39] DeGregorio, R., N. A. Fenske, and L. F. Glass, Granulomatous slack skin: a possible precursor of Hodgkin's disease. *J Am Acad Dermatol*, 1995. 33(6): p. 1044-7.

[40] Thein, M., et al., Syringotropic cutaneous T-cell lymphoma: an immunophenotypic and genotypic study of five cases. *Br J Dermatol*, 2004. 151(1): p. 216-26.

[41] Hitchcock, M. G., et al., Eccrine gland infiltration by mycosis fungoides. *Am J Dermatopathol*, 1996. 18(5): p. 447-53.

[42] Pileri, A., et al., Syringotropic mycosis fungoides: a rare variant of the disease with peculiar clinicopathologic features. *Am J Surg Pathol*, 2011. 35(1): p. 100-9.

[43] de Masson, A., et al., Syringotropic mycosis fungoides: clinical and histologic features, response to treatment, and outcome in 19 patients. *J Am Acad Dermatol*, 2014. 71(5): p. 926-34.

[44] Gallardo, F., et al., Cutaneous lymphomas showing prominent granulomatous component: clinicopathological features in a series of 16 cases. *J Eur Acad Dermatol Venereol*, 2009. 23(6): p. 639-47.

[45] Goodlad, J. and E. Calonje, Cutaneous lymphoproliferative diseases and related disorders. in *McKee's pathology of the skin: with clinical correlations*, E. Calonje, et al., Editors. 2012, Elsevier/Saunders: Edinburgh.

[46] Pankratov, O., et al., Poikilodermatous mycosis fungoides: clinical and histopathological analysis of a case and literature review. *Acta Dermatovenerol Alp Pannonica Adriat*, 2015. 24(2): p. 37-41.

[47] Kreuter, A., K. Hoffmamm, and P. Altmeyer, A case of poikiloderma vasculare atrophicans, a rare variant of cutaneous T-cell lymphoma, responding to extracorporeal photopheresis. *J Am Acad Dermatol*, 2005. 52(4): p. 706-8.

[48] Farley-Loftus, R., R. Mandal, and J. A. Latkowski, Poikilodermatous mycosis fungoides. *Dermatol Online J*, 2010. 16(11): p. 8.

[49] Bloom, B., et al., Poikilodermatous mycosis fungoides. *Dermatol Online J*, 2012. 18(12): p. 4.

[50] Patraquim, C., et al., Childhood Hypopigmented Mycosis Fungoides: A Rare Diagnosis. *Case Rep Pediatr*, 2016. 2016: p. 8564389.

[51] Rodney, I. J., et al., Hypopigmented mycosis fungoides: a retrospective clinicohistopathologic study. *J Eur Acad Dermatol Venereol*, 2016.

[52] Furlan, F. C., et al., Hypopigmented mycosis fungoides versus mycosis fungoides with concomitant hypopigmented lesions: same disease or different variants of mycosis fungoides? *Dermatology*, 2014. 229(3): p. 271-4.

[53] Soughi, M. and F. Z. Mernissi, Hyperpigmented mycosis fungoides: a rare variant. *Pan Afr Med J*, 2013. 15: p. 13.

[54] Xu, X. L., et al., Bullous mycosis fungoides: report of a case complicated by Kaposi's varicelliform eruption. *J Dermatol,* 2013. 40(10): p. 844-7.

[55] Bowman, P. H., D. J. Hogan, and I. D. Sanusi, Mycosis fungoides bullosa: report of a case and review of the literature. *J Am Acad Dermatol*, 2001. 45(6): p. 934-9.

[56] Inchara, Y. K. and T. Rajalakshmi, Early mycosis fungoides vs. inflammatory mimics: how reliable is histology? *Indian J Dermatol Venereol Leprol*, 2008. 74(5): p. 462-6.

[57] Santucci, M., et al., Efficacy of histologic criteria for diagnosing early mycosis fungoides: an EORTC cutaneous lymphoma study group investigation. European Organization for Research and Treatment of Cancer. *Am J Surg Pathol,* 2000. 24(1): p. 40-50.

[58] Beswick, T. C. and J. B. Cohen, Dose-related levetiracetam-induced reticulated drug eruption. *J Drugs Dermatol,* 2010. 9(4): p. 409-10.

[59] Mutasim, D. F., Lymphomatoid drug eruption mimicking digitate dermatosis: cross reactivity between two drugs that suppress angiotensin II function. *Am J Dermatopathol*, 2003. 25(4): p. 331-4.

[60] Hession, M. T. and P. L. Scheinman, Lymphomatoid allergic contact dermatitis mimicking cutaneous T cell lymphoma. *Dermatitis,* 2010. 21(4): p. 220.

[61] Knackstedt, T. J. and K. A. Zug, T cell lymphomatoid contact dermatitis: a challenging case and review of the literature. *Contact Dermatitis*, 2015. 72(2): p. 65-74.

In: Mycosis Fungoides and Sézary Syndrome ISBN: 978-1-68507-093-9
Editors: X. Zhang and L. Sokol

Chapter 4

Pathological Features of Mycosis Fungoides with Large Cell Transformation

Pukhraz Basra*[1]*, MD,
Priyatharsini Nirmalanantham*[1]*, MD
and Ling Zhang*[2,*]*, MD
[1]University Hospitals Cleveland Medical Center
Cleveland, OH, USA
[2]H. Lee Moffitt Cancer Center and Research Institute
Tampa, FL, USA

Introduction

Although patients with mycosis fungoides (MF) typically experience an indolent disease course, a minority undergo a process of large-cell transformation (LCT), which often heralds a more aggressive clinical course and shortened survival. LCT of MF is defined as the presence of more than

* Corresponding Author's Email: ling.zhang@moffitt.org.

25% large cells within the atypical lymphoid infiltrate. The transformed cells are invariably large T cells with cerebriform or indented nuclei. Immunophenotypically, LCT of MF cells are CD3+ and CD4+ with a frequent loss of CD5, CD2 and/or CD7, similar to the pre-transformed MF component. Co-expression of CD30 is identified in a subpopulation of patients (30-50%) and can also be found in small T-cells in conventional MF, therefore, CD30 is not considered a reliable marker for recognition of LCT. Clinically, 20-50% of LCT occurs usually at the phase of disease progression, however, LCT can present as an initial manifestation of MF. Indolent LCT has also been observed [17]. Transformed MF at the time of the initial diagnosis may carry a better prognosis compared to transformed MF cases diagnosed in the late disease course [3]. Poor prognostic factors in LCT include advanced clinical stage, early onset of transformation (defined as less than 2 years from the time of initial MF diagnosis), extracutaneous site involvement, high proliferation index measured by Ki67 immunostaining, and elevated β-2 microglobulin and lactate dehydrogenase (LDH) level.

LCT has classically been described as occurring within MF tumor lesions. A recent study identified 3 clinical patterns of LCT in MF patients: (1) a new solitary nodule within a long-standing classic MF patch/plaque, (2) the abrupt onset of multiple nodules that persist, and (3) a new or enlarging tumor [3].

There is a paucity of information in the reported literature concerning the LCT risk factors for patients with Sézary syndrome (SS) due to its low incidence. However, given the generally poor prognosis associated with this transformation, there is a need to reveal the associated factors and assess the risk of LCT before it is diagnosed. Although studies have shown that MF and LCT have a common clonal origin, the morphologic, phenotypic, and molecular risk factors that result in the development of LCT are largely unknown [11].

It is paramount for clinicians to be able to recognize suspicious lesions, as the diagnosis of LCT typically triggers more aggressive therapy and/or referral to cutaneous T-cell lymphoma (CTCL) centers. The distinction of LCT of MF vs. primary cutaneous anaplastic large cell lymphoma (C-

ALCL) as well as other T cell lymphomas, based on clinical-pathological correlation, is also extremely important since the two entities differ greatly in clinical outcome and treatment strategies.

PATHOLOGICAL DIAGNOSIS

Morphology

Microscopic review of a punch biopsy of skin shows increased (> 25%) large atypical lymphoid cells, defined as > 4× the size of a small lymphocyte in the dermal infiltrates or forming microscopic nodules [18-19]. These cells have cerebriform or indented nuclei and microscopically often form clusters or masses associated with the background of small-to-medium sized atypical lymphoid cells with or without epidermotropism (Fig. 4-1). Folliculotropism is identified in 1/3 of LCT cases [19].

LCT usually involves superficial dermis or deep down to papillary dermis with or without association with intravascular involvement, and dermal fibrosis [3].

LCT can manifest with enlarged regional lymph nodes or circulating large atypical forms. A biopsy of the lymph node can show focal, partial or full effacement of nodal architecture with interfollicular expansion of increased large atypical T-cells. It is often associated with overt dermatopathic changes due to skin irritation which may mask a low-level involvement by MF. Peripheral blood morphologic findings cannot separate them from *de novo* Sézary syndrome (SS).

Immunophenotyping

The morphology of large cells ranges from enlarged round or slightly oval, vesicular nuclei and scant cytoplasm to cells with large oval vesicular nuclei, large nucleoli, and abundant cytoplasm, making this entity indistinguishable from C-ALCL when a clear history of MF is not evident.

CTLC with large cell transformation

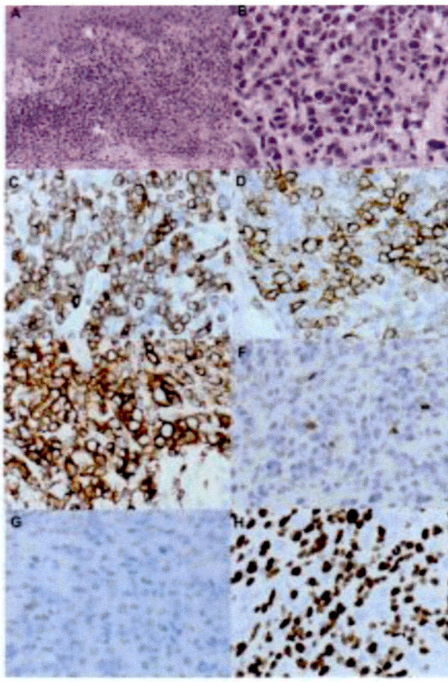

Figure 4-1. A-B. Medium to high power review of skin biopsy shows subepidermal dense atypical lymphoid infiltrate with increased large atypical forms displaying convoluted nuclear contour, disperse chromatin and come with conspicuous nucleoli (H&E x 200, B H&E x 600), C-H. A panel of immunohistochemical stains highlight the neoplastic cells to be positive for CD3 (C. immunoperoxidase, x 600), CD30 (D. Immunoperoxidase, x 600), CD4 (E. immunoperoxidase, x600), and negative for CD8 and CD7 (F and G. Immunoperoxidase, x600) with high proliferation index (estimated Ki67 of 80%) (H. Immunoperoxidase, x600).

Flow cytometry or immunohistochemistry studies can be applied for the diagnosis. Immunophenotypically, LCT of MF cells are CD3+ and CD4+ with a frequent loss of CD7 and CD26 and a loss of CD5, CD2 and/or CD7, similar to the pre-transformed MF component. Additionally, CD25 expression can be seen. Although small and large B cells are often prominent in infiltrates of transformed MF, as reactive features, aberrant CD20 expression has also been confirmed on the surface of the neoplastic T cells [3]. By immunohistochemical staining, the MF cells show similar immunophenotype as identified by flow cytometry. The transformed tumor cells are typically CD4+, although they may acquire a cytotoxic phenotype with the expression of cytotoxic molecules such as TIA-1, perforin, and granzyme B.

The expression of CD30 (Ki-1), a marker of lymphocyte activation, in some cases of LCT suggests a shift to an activating phenotype [17]. Some degree of CD30 expression is seen in 30–50% of cases, and in half of these, ≥ 75% of the infiltrate expresses this antigen. In general, when mixed with fewer than 75% CD30+ large T cells, a diagnosis of transformed MF is favored over diagnoses of primary C-ALCL [2]. When more than 75% of large cells are CD30+, it could be difficult to distinguish between these entities and transformed MF on histology alone without clear clinical information. Of note, the CD30+ T cells identified in pre-transformed stage are usually small or medium in size. Therefore, it is important to highlight that the expression of CD30 should *not* be used as a marker of transformation.

Recent studies have emerged with immunohistochemical markers to help with the diagnosis of LCT of MF, including GATA-3 and p53. Overexpression of GATA-3, a regulator of Th2 differentiation, may favor MF with LCT over ALCL as the latter tends to be negative for this marker [5, 33]. p53 overexpression has been correlated with the transformation, but this is not associated with a *TP53* gene mutation and is of uncertain significance [6]. Further research is required to determine the absolute utility of these markers in the setting of LCT of MF.

Molecular Genetics

Although studies have shown that MF and LCT have a common clonal origin, the morphologic, phenotypic, and molecular risk factors that result in the development of LCT are largely unknown [2, 7, 8].

More recently, loss of CDKN2A/CDKN2B as well as overexpression of micro-RNAs miR-93-5p, miR-181a, miR181b, miR-34a, and miR-326 have been documented at high frequency in LCT of MF, but the role these abnormalities play in disease progression remains undetermined [9,10].

DIFFERENTIAL DIAGNOSIS

LCT of MF should show morphologic and immunophenotypic overlapping with a list of following diseases, primary or secondary cutaneous involvements which include lymphomatoid papulosis (LyP) and C-ALCL. A consensus was reached by using a diagnostic algorithm to distinguish between LCT of MF and other diseases, using three features: large cell lymphoma cytology, pre-existing MF, and CD30 antigen expression by large cells [32] (Fig. 4-2).

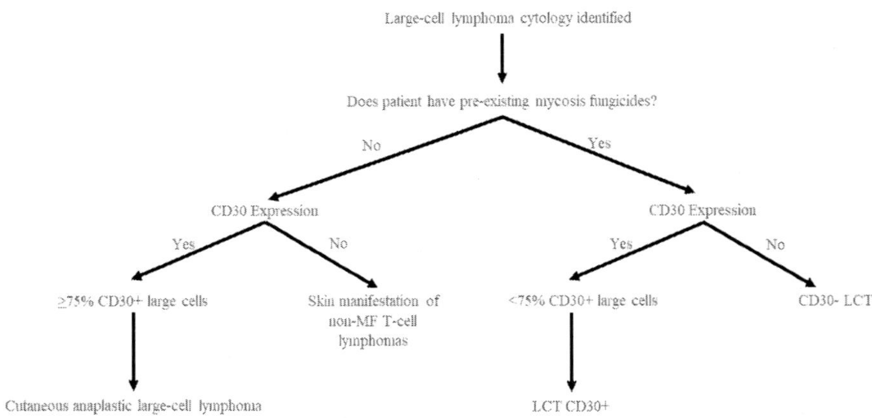

Figure 4-2. US Cutaneous Lymphoma Consortium algorithm for classification of skin tumors in patients with cutaneous T-cell lymphoma, using three features: large cell lymphoma cytology, pre-existing mycosis fungoides, and CD30 antigen expression by large cells.

It is crucial to distinguish CD30+ LCT from LyP and C-ALCL which may also develop in patients with MF (especially LyP). Clinical course is often the only distinguishing feature among both conditions [3]. The observation that MF and another CD30+ lymphoproliferative disorder, LyP, can coexist, introduces the concept that Lyp and C-ALCL represent two ends of a clinicopathologic continuum of CD30+ cutaneous lymphoproliferative disorders [7, 8].

Lymphomatoid Papulosis

Different from LCT, LyP is an indolent cutaneous lymphoproliferative disorder with waxing and waning clinical course lasting years to decades. It shows heterogeneous histologic patterns (A-F) that can be subcategorized into 6 variants with variable degree of CD30 co-expression. Morphologically, LyP type B lesions could mimic MF but are associated with papular lesion that could regress spontaneously. The type C lesions show collections of large atypical CD30+ cells and less inflammatory cells in the background. It resembles C-ALCL or MF with LCT. Clinical presentation is key in distinguishing between type C LyP and MF with LCT.

A variant of LyP with folliculocentric pattern of growth was reported and called "type F" by some. These lesions may be confused with folliculitis and eosinophilic folliculitis. Cases of LyP harboring chromosomal rearrangements of the *DUSP22-IRF4* locus on 6p25.3 have been recently reported. These lesions reveal a biphasic pattern of growth with large cells in deeper portions of the infiltrate and small cells involving the epidermis. CD30 labeling also follows a biphenotypic pattern. Distinction from more aggressive processes, such as MF with LCT, is again greatly helped by the clinical presentation of recurrent and self-healing papules and nodules [20].

Cutaneous ALCL

C-ALCL is currently defined as a cutaneous tumor of large cells with anaplastic, pleomorphic or immunoblastic morphology that express the CD30 antigen by the majority (75%) of tumor cells [2]. According to the World Health Organization Classification of Tumors of Hematopoietic and Lymphoid Tissues, patients with primary C-ALCL should not have clinical evidence or a history of MF [9]. LCT of MF is frequently diagnosed in the setting of a patient with a known history of MF while patients with C-ALCL may lack such a history.

To date, no reliable criteria for the distinction of C-ALCL and LCT complicating MF have been developed. About 40% of CD30+ large-cell lymphoma (LCT) skin lesions arising in patients with MF have more than 75% large cells. The other 60% contain a polymorphous mixture including small cerebriform cells and intermediate types as well as large cells. Therefore, most CD30 + MF-LCT cases can be distinguished from C-ALCL on this basis alone. Second, about one-third of cases of CD30+ MF-LCT show folliculotropism by small cerebriform cells, whereas this has not been appreciated in C-ALCL. Third, CD30+ large-cell lymphoma lesions that develop in patients with prior or simultaneous lesions of patch/plaque MF are believed to represent MF-LCT, rather than C-ALCL. Finally, anaplastic lymphoma kinase (ALK) expression may only infrequently be helpful in making the distinction between C-ALCL and MF-LCT because ALK is rarely expressed in C-ALCL, often in a cytoplasmic-only distribution, and not at all in MF-LCT [2].

Adult T-Cell Lymphoma/Leukemia, Cutaneous Manifestation

Adult T-cell leukemia/lymphoma (ATLL) is a peripheral T-cell lymphoma resulting from infection with human T-cell lymphotropic virus-1 (HTLV-1). More than 50% of these patients have cutaneous involvement making skin the most common site of involvement, after peripheral blood [23]. Chronic and smoldering variants often present with patches, plaques and papular skin lesions, which may closely resemble MF, and circulating neoplastic T cells are few or absent [25]. The patients can present with skin-first at the time of presentation, or at some point during their clinical course. Of note, more than 80% of ATLL patients in the United States have misdiagnosis of CTCL, due to its rarity and its clinicopathologic mimicry of primary CTCLs, such as MF and systemic T-cell lymphoma. Delayed diagnosis of ATLL has negative impact on patient's survival [24].

The skin lesions of ATLL range from an exfoliative rash to papules and nodules, and some with ulceration [23]. The purely cutaneous form of the disease presents with erythematopapular and tumoral lesions, resembling that of MF. The diagnosis of ATLL in the United States should be considered with the following features [22, 23]:

1. Living in or coming from an HTLV-1 endemic region
2. Features of MF/SS with prominent pautrier-like microabcesses with large cell morphology
3. Nodulotumoral skin lesions presenting earlier than expected for CTCL
4. Cutaneous lesions not consistent with another well-recognized lymphoma
5. Expression of mature T-cell markers CD2, CD5, CD25 (strong and uniform), CD4/CD8 ratio > 10:1, loss of CD7, and expression of CCR4 and PD-1 [21, 22].

Peripheral T-Cell Lymphoma, NOS

Primary cutaneous peripheral T-cell lymphoma, NOS (PTCL, NOS) is the rarest form of CTCL and is a diagnosis of exclusion, with an aggressive and life-threatening consequence that often manifests with plaque-like skin lesions, generalized, or solitary/localized tumors [26]. Rapid progression of the cutaneous tumors and systemic involvement are key features of primary PTCL, NOS, making prompt diagnosis critical [25, 26]. Different from MF with LCT, polymorphous cell population with histiocytes, eosinophils, plasma cells, and heterogeneous population of lymphocytes have been reported in 70% of cases [26]. The immunophenotype of this entity varies, but most cases are CD4+ T cells with variable loss of pan-T cell antigens, limited or absent CD30 and rarely CD56 co-expression [25, 26], which makes the diagnosis challenging. Secondary skin involvement by systemic PTCL, NOS, can be determined in accordance with prior lymph node biopsy and clinical course.

Angioimmunoblastic T-Cell Lymphoma, Cutaneous Form

In angioimmunoblastic T-cell lymphoma (AITL), patients present with generalized lymphadenopathy, hepatosplenomegaly, high fever, night sweats, and weight loss, along with findings of hemolytic anemia, leukocytosis, and polyclonal hypergammaglobulinemia. AITL is an aggressive disease with primary nodal involvement but about one-half of patients develop cutaneous eruption, either as the presenting sign or over the course of the disease, which typically appear as macule and papule distributed diffusely over the trunck and extremities, mimicking a viral exanthema, drug hypersensitivity reaction or MF. The cell of origin of AITL is the follicular helper T-cell expressing CD10, BCL-6, PD1, CXCL13, and ICOS, which is unique and can be a diagnostic clue. Other CTCL coexpress these markers are primary CD4+ small medium T-cell lymphoproliferative disorder. Clinical history and clinical suspicion for AITL becomes important. Immunophenotypically, the cutaneous lesion demonstrates T-cell phenotype with CD2, CD3, CD5 and intact CD7 and the aforementioned follicular T-helper markers, and predominance of CD4 + T-cells, distinguishing it from MF with LCT [27].

Leukemic Cutis/Monocytic Sarcoma

Leukemic cutis is defined by cutaneous lesions that are a result of the infiltration by neoplastic leukocytes (myeloid or lymphoid). Leukemic cutis is more commonly found in patients with acute myeloid leukemia (10-15%) [28], specifically, acute myelomonocytic (AMMoL) and monocytic (AMoL) types. In patients with chronic hematological diseases, the skin lesions represent transformation to blastic phase and disease progression [28]. Patients most commonly present with single or multiple lesions of erythematous papules and nodules [28]. The lesions with monocytic differentiation are often positive for CD4 and CD43 that could mimic T-cell processing. A history of myeloid leukemia/neoplasm, a rapidly eruption of skin lesions, and expression of CD68, CD163, lysozyme or MPO, are helpful to differentiate it from MF with LCT [28].

Cutaneous Involvement by Other Mature and Immature T-Cell Lymphoma/Leukemias

Leukemia cutis resulting from mature T-cell leukemias mainly includes three differentials: adult T-cell leukemia, T-cell prolymphocytic leukemia (T-PLL), and SS [28]. The neoplastic cells commonly express CD4 amongst the aforementioned three differentials, in addition to other immunophenotype characteristic of leukemic infiltrate, such as strong CD25+, CD4+, HTLV1+ for ATLL marked leukocytosis, hepatosplenomegaly, immunostaining positive for T-cell leukemia -1 (TCL-1), inv(14) or t(14;14) for T-PLL, rapidly diffuse erythematic skin lesion for *de novo* SS etc. Rarely, cutaneous T-ALL could occur, which usually manifests with immature precursor T-cells positive for CD1a, TdT and/or CD34.

Blastic Plasmacytoid Dendritic Cell Neoplasm

Blastic plasmacytoid dendritic cell neoplasm (BPDCN) is an aggressive rare malignancy with poor prognosis which should be easily separated from MF with LCT by distinct clinical manifestation (dark purple nodules to patches) and the following immunophenotype. BPDCN is derived from precursor plasmacytoid dendritic cells that express CD4, CD56, and ≥ 1 dendritic cell-associated antigens such as CD123, TCL1, blood dendritic cell antigen-2 (BDCA2/CD303), and TCF1, and negative for certain lineage-specific markers for myeloid cells (myeloperoxidase), T cells (CD3), B cells (CD20, PAX5, and CD79a), and monocytes (CD11c, CD163, lysozyme) and CD34. CD30 is usually negative. About 89% of BPDCN patients present with cutaneous lesions, followed by systemic dissemination [29].

Clinical Features

Clinical Course

It is paramount for clinicians to be able to recognize suspicious lesions, as the diagnosis of LCT typically triggers more aggressive therapy and/or referral to CTCL centers. The distinction of LCT of MF vs. C-ALCL based on clinical-pathological correlation, is also extremely important since the two entities differ greatly in prognosis. Large studies have shown the lack of evidence to support the role of viral infections or other environmental exposures in the pathogenesis of LCT. It is possible, however, that a causative external agent has not yet been identified [2].

MF is typically stratified by stage, which is based on extent of body surface area involvement, type of skin lesions, or presence of extra-cutaneous involvement in accordance with the International Society for Cutaneous Lymphomas (ISCL) and the European Organization for Research and Treatment (EORTC). LCT has been documented to occur in all stages of CTCL. However, it is most frequently diagnosed in patients with more advanced disease [4]. Arulogun et al. [8] found that in a cohort of 22 patients, only 1.4% of patients with early-stage disease developed LCT, whereas more than 25% of patients with stage IIB disease and more than 50% with stage IV disease transformed. LCT is typically identified in cutaneous rather than extra-cutaneous sites, though the latter could occur. Early recognition of the clinical clues associated with LCT allows the dermatologist to diagnose this entity earlier and offer patients more aggressive management. LCT is most likely to occur in cutaneous tumors and small papules with an increased rate of disease progression. There is little published data to guide dermatologists as to what clinical signs to assess in the detection of LCT. In a patient with a history of MF, the following are three reported clinical instances that lead to suspect the diagnosis of LCT of MF:

1. Erythematous papules that could clinically be mistaken for a bite or bacterial furuncle.

2. An abrupt onset of multiple nodules with or without ulceration and within or distinct from MF plaques.
3. Presentation of a combination of nodules and tumors or tumors alone.

It is recommended that any patient with MF who develops new papules, even if they are small and innocuous-looking, should receive a biopsy to evaluate for LCT. Concurrent clinical lymphadenopathy should prompt a PET/CT scan and/or lymph node biopsy to evaluate for MF with nodal transformation. Bone marrow biopsies are not routinely performed in all patients with LCT but are considered for those with refractory, advanced-stage cases [3].

Risk Stratification/Prognosis

There is a paucity of information in the reported literature concerning the LCT risk factors for patients with SS due to its low incidence. However, given the generally poor prognosis associated with this transformation, there is a need to reveal the associated factors and assess the risk of LCT before it is diagnosed. This knowledge is essential to developing targeted therapies for these patients, and preventing the complications associated with the more aggressive disease course.

A recent study conducted by Jairath et al., suggests that there are clinical and pathologic factors that may predict the development of LCT. These included greater maximum total body surface area (TBSA) with identifiable disease, peak LDH level, presence of ulceration, Langerhans cell hyperplasia, and decreased absolute CD8+ cell count at the time of SS diagnosis and at the most recent blood draw. Furthermore, TBSA may be a surrogate for disease aggression, rather than a modifiable disease factor, that is correlated with LCT [11].

Overall, features to predict outcome in patients with transformed MF include advanced stage at transformation, increased extent of skin lesions, folliculotropism, and Ki67 and CD30 expression [4, 6, 16-19]. Specifically,

Diamandidou et al., [16] found that early transformation (< 2 years after diagnosis) and advanced stages (stage IIB or higher) were associated with poor prognosis. Benner et al., [4] collected 100 cases of MF with LCT and reported that CD30 negativity, folliculotropic MF, the extent of skin lesions, and extracutaneous transformation were all associated with a reduced disease-specific survival. Another study by Talpur et al., [7] reported poor prognosis in combination with advanced age, LCT at the time of initial diagnosis of MF, high levels of LDH, and < 10% CD30 expression.

Clinical Outcomes

LCT is associated with a mean 5-year survival of less than 20% [1]. The patients with an indolent disease course are associated with a longer-term survival [30]. Better survival has been reported among patients who present with transformation at diagnosis as compared to those who transform later on. Clinical features are key determinants of prognosis among MF with LCT patients. Age (> 60 years), stage III/IV, high serum LDH, absent papillary dermal involvement, follicular mucin at transformation, and the absence of fibrosis at transformation, are all factors associated with shorter survival time among MF with LCT patients. As such, assessment of the aforementioned clinical features can aid in the prognosis work-up for the patients [17].

Conclusion

In summary, an immediate biopsy should be performed in patients with history of MF who present with new erythematous papules, to address the possibility of LCT. Cytological features, history of MF, and expression of CD30 help in differentiating LCT of MF from other key differential diagnoses such as Lyp, C-ALCL, PTCL NOS, AITL, leukemic cutis, and BPDCN. Specifically, the presence of more than 25% large cells, together with fewer than 75% CD30+ large T cells, in the setting of pre-existing MF, favors the diagnosis of LCT of MF. Clinical presentation is key in the diagnosis and in the prognostication of LCT of MF. Specifically, age, serum LDH, presence/absence of fibrosis and stage are key prognostic indicators of LCT of MF.

REFERENCES

[1] Salhany K E, Cousar J B, Greer J P, et al. Transformation of cutaneous T cell lymphoma to large cell lymphoma. A clinicopathologic and immunologic study. *Am. J. Pathol.* 1988; 132: pp. 265-277.

[2] Herrmann J L, Hughey L C. Recognizing large-cell transformation of mycosis fungoides. *J. Am. Acad. Dermatol.* 2012; 67: pp. 665-672.

[3] Vergier B, de Muret A, Beylot-Barry M, et al. Transformation of mycosis fungoides: clinicopathological and prognostic features of 45 cases. French Study Group of Cutaneous Lymphomas. *Blood* 2000; 95: pp. 2212-2218.

[4] Benner M F, Jansen P M, Vermeer M H, et al. Prognostic factors in transformed mycosis fungoides: a retrospective analysis of 100 cases. *Blood* 2012; 119: pp. 1643-1649.

[5] Hsi A C, Lee S J, Rosman I S, Carson K R, Kelley A, Viele V, et al. Expression of helper T cell master regulators in inflammatory dermatoses and primary cutaneous T-cell lymphomas: diagnostic implications. *J. Am. Acad. Dermatol.* 2015;72:159–67.

[6] Li G, Chooack L, Wolfe J T, et al. Overexpression of p53 protein in cutaneous T cell lymphoma: relationship to large cell transformation and disease progression. *J. Invest. Dermatol.* 1998; 110: pp. 767-770.

[7] Talpur R, Sui D, Gangar P, et al. Retrospective analysis of prognostic factors in 187 cases of transformed mycosis fungoides. *Clin. Lymphoma Myeloma Leuk.* 2016;16:49–56.

[8] Arulogun S O, Prince H M, Ng J, et al. Long-term outcomes of patients with advanced-stage cutaneous T-cell lymphoma and large cell transformation. *Blood* 2008;112:3082-7.

[9] Nicolae-Cristea A R, Benner M F, Zoutman W H, et. al. *Br. J. Dermatol.* 2015; 172: pp. 784-788.

[10] Marosvari D, Teglasi V, Csala I, et. al. Altered microRNA expression in folliculotropic and transformed mycosis fungoides. *Pathol. Oncol. Res.* 2015; 21: pp. 821-825.

[11] Jairath N, Jairath R, Bardhi R, et al. (2020). *Clinicopathologic Risk Factors for the Large Cell Transformation of Sézary Syndrome.* doi:10.1101/2020.06.01.20119669.

[12] Cioplea, M., et al. Dendritic cell distribution in mycosis fungoides vs. inflammatory dermatosis and other T-cell skin lymphoma. *Oncol. Lett.*, 2019. 17(5): p. 4055-4059.

[13] Deguchi, M., et al. Comparison of the distribution and numbers of antigen-presenting cells among T-lymphocyte-mediated dermatoses: CD1a+, factor XIIIa+, and CD68+ cells in eczematous dermatitis, psoriasis, lichen planus and graft-versus-host disease. *Arch. Dermatol. Res.*, 2002. 294(7): p. 297-302.

[14] Lin, T., et al. Langerhans cell hyperplasia in the tumor stage of mycosis fungoides: A mimic of Langerhans cell histiocytosis. *Dermatol. Sin.*, 2011. 29(101): p. 101-105.

[15] Meissner K, Löning T, and Rehpenning W. Epidermal Langerhans cells and prognosis of patients with mycosis fungoides and Sézary syndrome. *In Vivo*, 1993. 7(3): p. 277-80.

[16] Diamandidou E, Colome-Grimmer M, Fayad L, et al. Transformation of mycosis fungoides/Sézary syndrome: clinical characteristics and prognosis. *Blood* 1998; 92: pp. 1150-1159.

[17] Pulitzer M, et al. Mycosis fungoides with large cell transformation: clinicopathological features and prognostic factors. *Pathology*, 2014. 46(7): p. 610-6.

[18] Swerdlow SH, et al. *WHO Classification of Tumours of Haematopoietic and Lymphoid Tissues.* Revised 4th edn, 385–402 (International Agency for Research on Cancer (IARC), 2017).

[19] Cerroni L, Rieger E, Hödl S, et al. Clinicopathologic and immunologic features associated with transformation of mycosis fungoides to large-cell lymphoma. *Am. J. Surg. Pathol.* 1992; 16: pp. 543-552.

[20] Karai L J, Kadin M E, Hsi E D, et al. Chromosomal rearrangements of 6p25.3 define a new subtype of lymphomatoid papulosis. *Am. J. Surg. Pathol.* 2013;37:1173–81.

[21] Rangoonwala H I, Cascella M. Peripheral T-Cell Lymphoma. In: *StatPearls [Internet].* Treasure Island (FL): StatPearls Publishing; 2021 Jan-. Available from: https://www.ncbi.nlm.nih.gov/books/NBK562301/.

[22] Parsi M, Go M S, Ahmed A. Leukemia Cutis. In: *StatPerals [Internet]* Treasure Island (FL): StatPearls Publishing; 2021 Jan-https://www.ncbi.nlm.nih.gov/books/NBK541136/.

[23] Tadashi Y and Elaine S J. Adult T-Cell Leukemia/Lymphoma. *Hematopathology*, Chapter 33, 619-629.e4.

[24] Cohen L, Chen P L, Zhang L, et al. Skin-first nodulotumoral adult T-cell lymphoma mimicking cutaneous T-cell lymphoma. *JAAD Case Rep.* 2019 Jul 31;5(8):650-652.

[25] Rein W. Cutaneous T-Cell Lymphoma. *Dermatology,* 120, 2127-2147.

[26] Aderhold K, Carpenter L, Brown K, et al. Primary Cutaneous Peripheral T-Cell Lymphoma Not Otherwise Specified: A Rapidly Progressive Variant of Cutaneous T-Cell Lymphoma. *Case Rep. Oncol. Med.* 2015;2015:429068.

[27] Jayaraman A G, Cassarino D, Advani R, et al. Cutaneous involvement by angioimmunoblastic T-cell lymphoma: a unique histologic presentation, mimicking an infectious etiology. *J. Cutan. Pathol.* 2006 Sep;33 Suppl 2:6-11.

[28] Cho-Vega J H, Medeiros L J, Prieto V G, et al. Leukemia cutis. *Am. J. Clin. Pathol.* 2008 Jan;129(1):130-42.

[29] Laribi K, Baugier de Materre A, Sobh M, et al. Blastic plasmacytoid dendritic cell neoplasms: results of an international survey on 398 adult patients. *Blood Adv.* 2020 Oct 13;4(19):4838-4848.

[30] Agar N S, Wedgeworth E, Crichton S, et al. Survival outcomes and prognostic factors in mycosis fungoides/Sézary syndrome: validation of the revised International Society for Cutaneous Lymphomas/

European Organisation for Research and Treatment of Cancer staging proposal. *J. Clin. Oncol.* 2010; 28:4730–9.

[31] Barberio E, Thomas L, Skowron F, et al. Transformed mycosis fungoides: clinicopathological features and outcome. *Br. J. Dermatol.* 2007 Aug;157(2):284-9.

[32] Kadin M E, Hughey L C, Wood G S. Large-cell transformation of mycosis fungoides-differential diagnosis with implications for clinical management: a consensus statement of the US Cutaneous Lymphoma Consortium. *J. Am. Acad. Dermatol.* 2014 Feb;70(2):374-6.

[33] Basra P, Gajzer D, Sokol L, et al. *GATA3 Expression and Ki67 Proliferation Index as Diagnostic Tools in Mycosis Fungoides and its Mimickers.* USCAP 2020 abstract. February 28-March 5, 2020. Los Angeles.

In: Mycosis Fungoides and Sézary Syndrome ISBN: 978-1-68507-093-9
Editors: X. Zhang and L. Sokol

Chapter 5

Histopathological Differential Diagnosis of Early Mycosis Fungoides with Benign Dermatoses

Jianping Cai**, MD
Dianon Systems/Laboratory Corporation of America,
Tampa, FL, USA

Introduction

Being the most common form of cutaneous T cell lymphoma, mycosis fungoides is usually presented as a slowly evolving indolent disease over many years and even decades, with most patients having a long-lasting history of patch or plaque lesions on sun-protected areas. Although the majority of patients with MF do not die of the disease, but rather die with the disease, the accurate diagnosis of early MF is still quite critical in terms of disease staging, prognostic evaluation, and decision-making for therapeutic options [1-3].

* Corresponding Author's Email: jianpingcai1963@gmail.com.

Histologic diagnosis of early MF (patch and early plaque stages of the disease) is probably one of the most challenging tasks in the field of dermatopathology, mainly because almost all the pathologic changes in early lesion of MF can variably occur in many benign inflammatory dermatoses [4, 5]. While clinical correlation plays a very important role in arriving at a timely histologic diagnosis of MF [6, 7], knowing the differential pathologic features of the various related benign dermatoses under the conventional microscopy, in combination with immunohistochemical staining for phenotyping, as well as molecular testing for clonality of the T cell receptor (TCR) gene rearrangement, could greatly increase the likelihood for the pathologist, the microscopic diagnostician, to achieve that goal [8, 9].

I like to start this chapter of the monograph by showing a few photomicrographs with diagnostic features of patch or plaque stage of MF. In these photos, one can appreciate the prominent lymphocytic epidermotropism with small lymphocytes scattered in the epidermis, and particularly lined along the basal layer of the epidermis forming the phenomenon called string of pearls (Figure 5-1A, B). In the papillary dermis there is fibrosis associated with infiltration of mononuclear cells (Figure 5-1A, B). In other sections, there is a quite dense superficial dermal lymphocytic infiltrate with very prominent epidermotropism in the epidermis, and on high power "atypical" lymphocytes with irregular nuclear contour displaying cerebriform nuclei can be seen in the epidermis (Figure 5-1C, D). Upon initial examination of the slides under light microscope, a pathologist may come up with a preliminary thought of histologic diagnosis of MF. After learning that the specimen was actually a re-excision for a biopsy-proven squamous cell carcinoma in situ, the pathologist realized that the observed histopathologic features diagnostic for MF were merely the tissue reaction of host to the previous biopsy procedure. In my 16 years of practice of dermatopathology of large daily volume, I have observed quite often this type of "diagnostic histologic features of MF" associated with re-excision specimens. I put out this example to illustrate how vitally important the clinical correlation should play in the histopathologic diagnosis of early stage MF. One may certainly make an incorrect diagnosis of MF if only based on histopathologic features of a particular case.

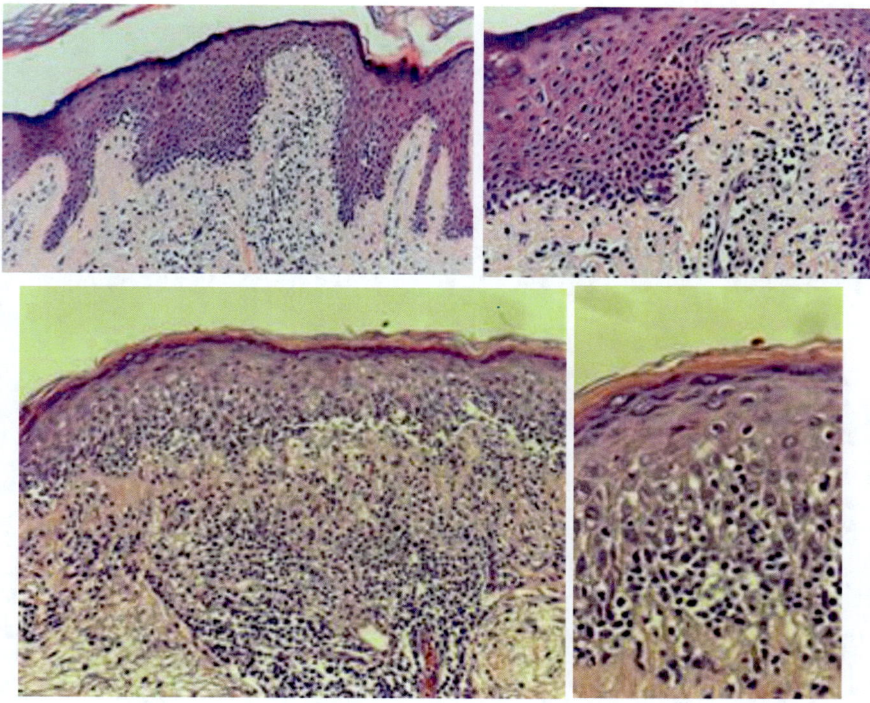

Figure 5-1. Re-excision specimen for SCC in situ mimicking MF. A (top left) & B (top right): prominent epidermotropism with lymphocytes lining up along the basal layers of the epidermis. C (bottom left): dense dermal lymphocytic infiltrate with epidermotropism. D (bottom right): high power view showing irregular nuclear contour of epidermotropic "atypical" lymphocytes with halos.

Before we start to go into details for the differential histopathologic diagnosis of early MF with individual entity of benign dermatoses, it is important to first review the fundamental features that are very helpful in making histologic diagnosis of early MF [10-15]: Pautrier microabscesses (Figure 5-2B, C), epidermotropism of lymphocytes, particularly with lymphocytes aligning along the basal layer of epidermis (Figure 5-2A), intraepidermal lymphocytes with a clear perinuclear halo (Figure 5-2A), intraepidermal lymphocytes with hyperchromatic and convoluted nuclei, and intraepidermal lymphocytes with nuclei larger than the nuclei of dermal infiltrating lymphocytes.

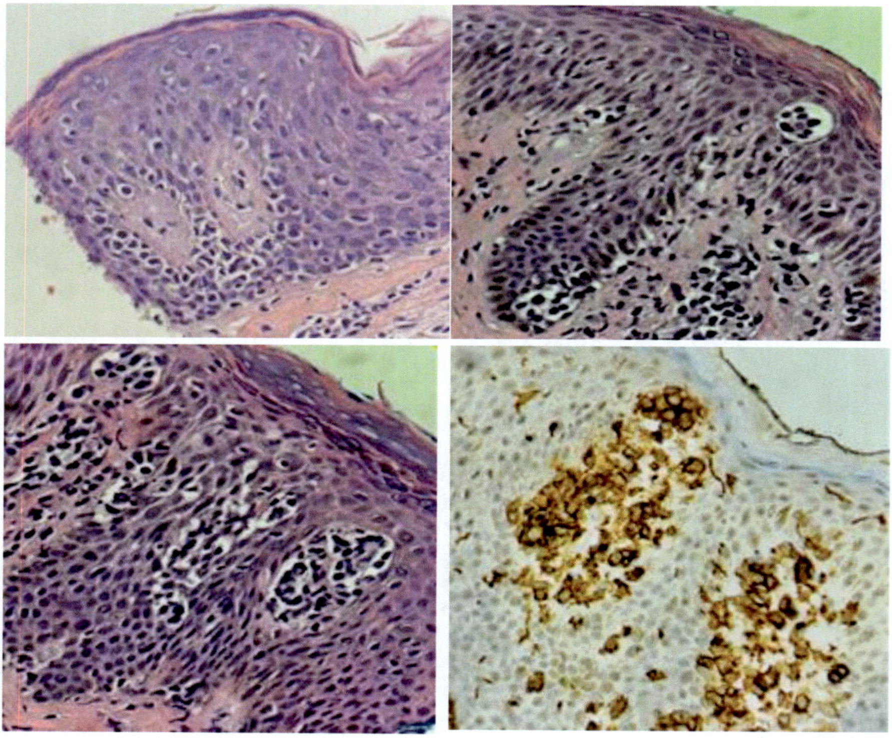

Figure 5-2. Early patch stage MF. A (top left): epidermotropic lymphocytes aligne along the basal layer of epidermis with appearance of string of pearls. B (top right) & C (bottom left): collections of lymphocytes in epidermis forming Pautrier's microabcesses. D (bottom right): CD4 immunostain.

In the following paragraphs, the salient key histologic features of the individual entities of benign inflammatory dermatoses, which are useful in differentiating them from early stage of MF, will be discussed, with particular mentioning of some aspects of their presentation resembling MF. It will cover three main categories of different histologic patterns of inflammatory dermatoses, namely spongiotic dermatitis, interface/lichenoid dermatitis, and psoriasiform dermatitis.

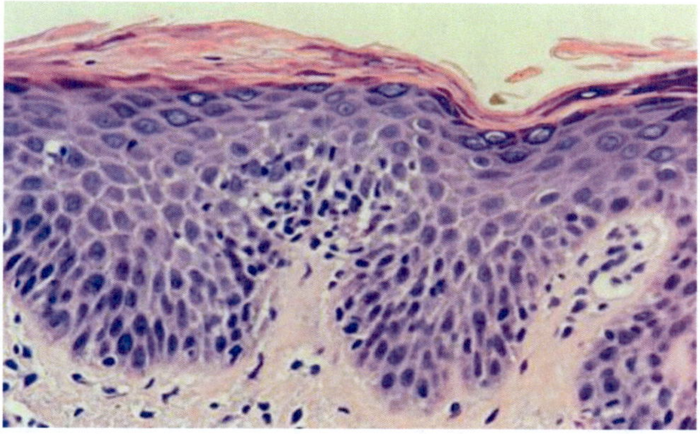

Figure 5-3. Chronic superficial dermatitis. Acanthosis with mild epidermal spongiosis, and sparse superficial perivascular lymphocytic infiltrate focally extending upward into the epidermis (exocytosis).

SPONGIOTIC DERMATITIS

Chronic Superficial Dermatitis (Small Plaque Parapsoriasis, Digitate Dermatosis)

This condition is featured clinically by oval to round, well-defined, patches, sometimes with fine "cigarette-paper" appearance. The onset is usually at middle age with a male predominance. Most chronic superficial dermatitis will not progress to CTCL. Although histologically it is usually classified in the category of spongiotic dermatitis tissue reaction pattern, epidermal spongiosis is mild and focal, with mild epidermal acanthosis. Psoriasiform epidermal hyperplasia is rare and may only occur in older lesions with chronic irritation. A very sparse superficial perivascular lymphocytic infiltrate is usually present. This mild lymphocytic infiltrate may extend upward into the epidermis very focally (exocytosis) [16]. As we can see from the above description, the histologic features of chronic superficial dermatosis are entirely non-specific, and clinical correlation is crucial in reaching the correct diagnosis for this particular condition. The key histologic features that can be used to exclude this from early MF are the lack of prominent lymphocytic epidermotropism and the lack of atypia in lymphocytes.

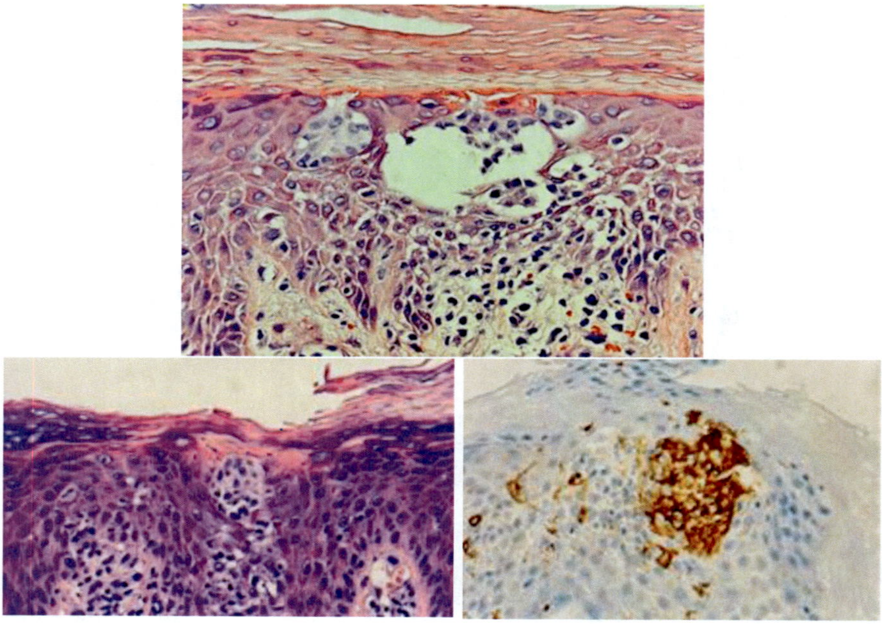

Figure 5-4. Subacute/chronic spongiotic dermatitis. A (top) & B (bottom left): epidermal spongiosis with collections of Langerhans cells in the epidermis. C (bottom right): CD1a immunostain.

Subacute and Chronic Spongiotic Dermatitis

The tissue reaction pattern of subacute and chronic spongiotic dermatitis can be seen in a group of various eczematous dermatitides that include the clinical entities of allergic contact dermatitis, nummular dermatitis, atopic dermatitis, and seborrheic dermatitis. With progressing chronicity, the spongiosis will subside, and epidermal psoriasiform hyperplasia will gradually become more evident, even taking the form to the degree of lichen simplex chronicus, coupled with mild papillary dermal fibrosis.

The acute form of spongiotic dermatitis rarely presents a diagnostic challenge histopathologically, particularly not a consideration for differentiating from MF because of prominent spongiosis, and sometimes with intraepidermal microvesiculation, associated with "wet" appearance with surface scale crust. In the epidermis, lymphocytic exocytosis can be marked with conspicuous epidermal Langerhans cells and other inflammatory cells forming microabscesses resembling Pautrier's microabscesses in MF (Figure 5-4A and B). Usually this type of intraepidermal collection of Langerhans cells and other inflammatory cells takes the shape of flask, with the mouth of the flask opening at the stratum corneum [17]. Immunostain of CD1a positivity of such collection of cells can confirm the Langerhans cell nature of the microabscesses (Figure 5-4C).

In subacute and chronic spongiotic dermatitis, it occasionally can be quite challenging to differentiate from MF histopathologically [18, 19], when lymphocytic exocytosis is prominent (Figure 5-5A and B), and even with intraepidermal lymphocytes tagging along the basal layer (Figure 5A). Lymphocyte exocytosis proportionate to the degree of spongiosis is helpful in favoring the diagnosis of subacute spongiotic dermatitis. Immunostains showing mixed CD4 and CD8 positive T cells in the intraepidermal lymphocytic population can also aid in the diagnosis as shown in Figure 5-5C and D.

INTERFACE/LICHENOID DERMATITIS

Lichen Planus

Lichen planus has quite specific histopathologic features that would allow one to render a definitive diagnosis in most cases, so it rarely presents a diagnostic challenge to the dermatopathologists, usually not into play for the said diagnostic confusion with MF. But the dense band-like lichenoid mononuclear cell infiltrate seen in lichen planus, particularly if combined with prominent lymphocytic exocytosis at the dermoepidermal junction, can occasionally put MF on the list of differential diagnoses [20, 21]. In this particular setting, there are usually sufficient and multiple other distinctive histologic features diagnostic for lichen planus that can aid in the exclusion of MF.

Lichen planus usually shows acanthosis that is irregular and often times with a sawtooth appearance. There is wedge-shaped hypergranulosis which is quite unique for lichen planus (Figure 5-6A). The chronic lichenoid lymphohistiocytic inflammatory host response can result in a prominent basal cell layer hydropic degeneration as well as focal squamatization. One can usually see few or many dyskeratotic keratinocytes along the basal cell layer and above it (so-called "Civatte" or "colloid" bodies). Additionally, unlike in MF, plasma cells and eosinophils are usually absent in lichen planus. Lichen planus usually shows pigment incontinence with scattered melanophages in the papillary dermis.

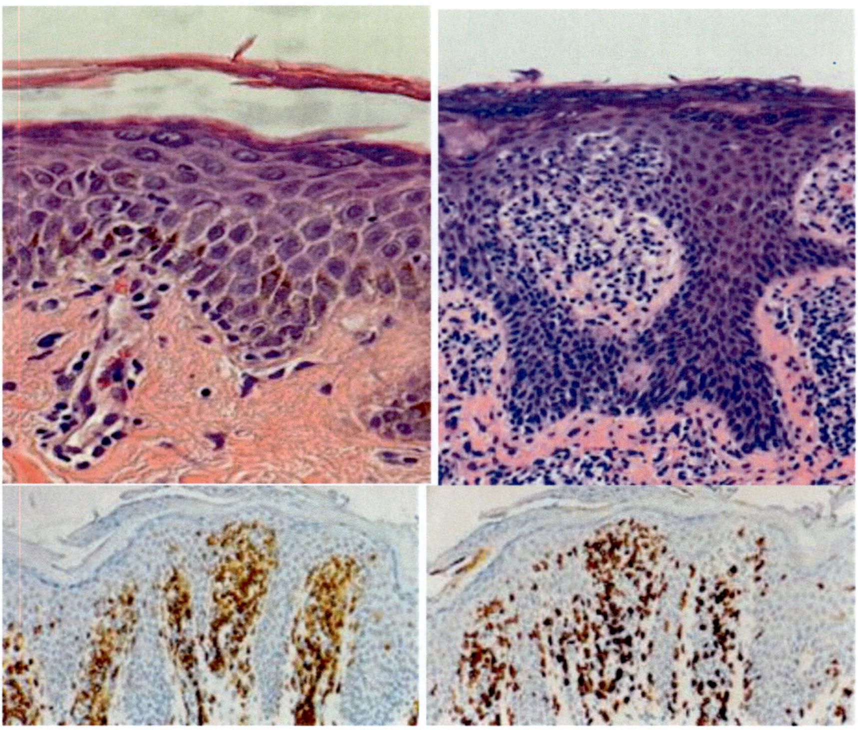

Figure 5-5. Subacute/chronic spongiotic dermatitis. A (top left): lymphocytes lining up along the basal layer of epidermis with the appearance of so-called "string of pearls," with mild to moderate degree of spongiosis. B (top right): moderately dense superficial dermal lymphocytic infiltrate with exocytosis of small lymphocytes in the epidermis forming small aggregates. C (bottom left): CD4 immunostain. D (bottom right): CD8 immunostain.

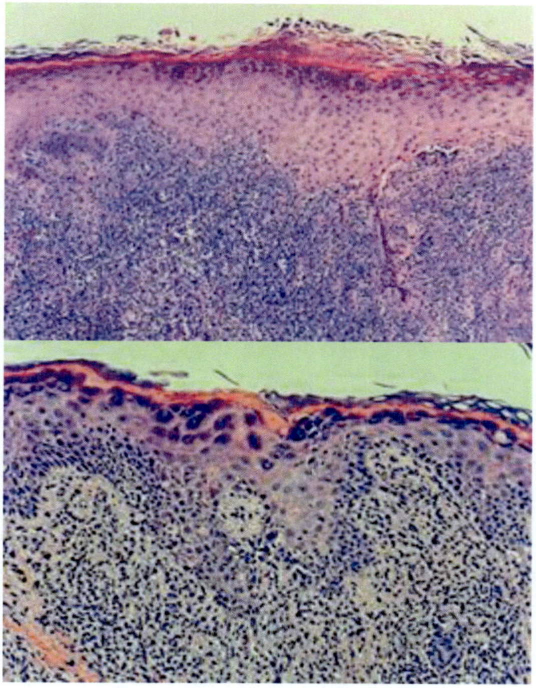

Figure 5-6. Lichen planus. A (top): extremely dense superficial dermal lymphocytic infiltrate, and irregular acanthosis with a sawtooth appearance, and wedge-shaped hypergranulosis. B (bottom): pigment incontinence with melanophages in the dermis.

Lichen Planus-Like Keratosis

The most frequent clinical differential diagnosis that accompanies a biopsy of lichen planus-like keratosis (LPLK) is probably basal cell carcinoma. That clinical information can be used in support of the diagnosis of LPLK, especially with cases showing histologic features mimicking MF. Since clinical indication of BCC points to a solitary lesion, and except in very rare cases of unilesional MF, MF usually presents as multiple lesions or diffuse skin condition.

It is not very uncommon that suspicion for the diagnosis of MF is raised when LPLK presents histologically with dense band-like superficial dermal lymphoid infiltrate, in combination with epidermal exocytosis of lymphocytes, sometimes in alignment along the basilar epidermis, with extension into the lower portion of the epidermis [17, 22]. Features that are helpful in favor of LPLK are the interface/florid lichenoid tissue reaction pattern resulting in prominent hydropic degeneration of the dermo-epidermal junction with variable numbers of dyskeratotic keratinocytes noted, focal wedge-shaped hypergranulosis, although usually less pronounced than in lichen planus, a contiguous adjacent solar lentigo or large cell acanthoma, or incipient seborrheic keratosis [17].

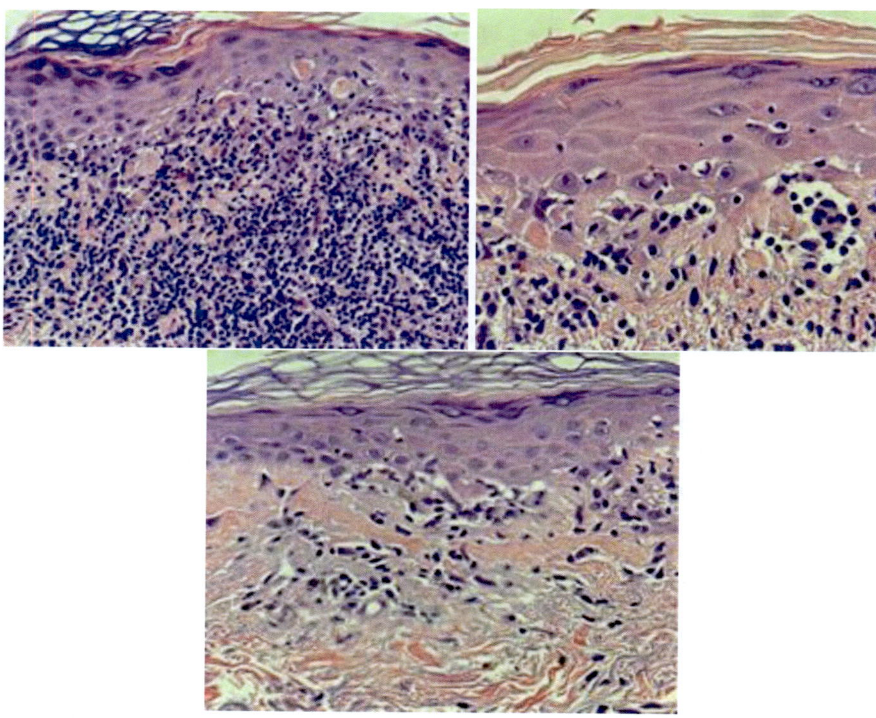

Figure 5-7. Lichen planus-like keratosis. A (top left): dense band-like superficial dermal lymphocytic infiltrate with interface reaction changes and many dyskeratotic keratinocytes. B (top right) and C (bottom): lymphocytic exocytosis in the epidermis forming small aggregates.

Lichenoid Drug Eruption

Histologic features of dense band-like lichenoid inflammatory infiltrate with lymphocytic exocytosis in the epidermis in lichenoid drug eruption can occasionally raise the consideration of MF for the pathologists. Besides the various histologic features mentioned in the paragraph below the heading of lichen planus that are usually also present in lichenoid drug eruption, there are several additional features that can further aid in reaching the diagnosis of lichenoid drug eruption (Figure 5-8). Parakeratosis is more frequently present in lichenoid drug eruption, and is a feature against the diagnosis of lichen planus. The presence of eosinophils favors the diagnosis of lichenoid drug eruption. Also, melanin pigment incontinence occurs relatively more often in lichenoid drug eruption.

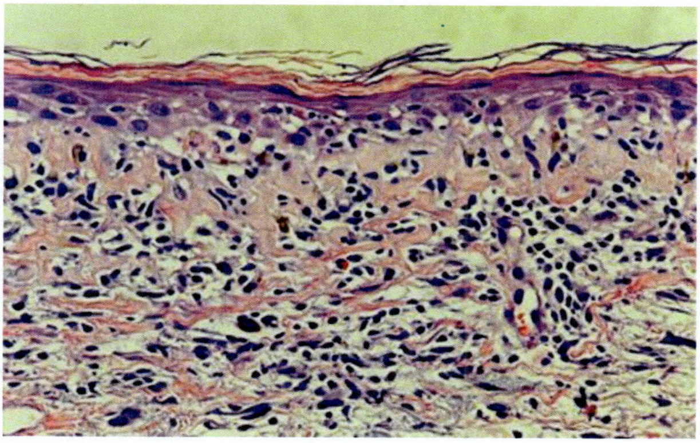

Figure 5-8. Lichenoid drug eruption. Relatively atrophic epidermis with prominent basal cell layer hydropic degeneration, moderately dense dermal lymphocytic infiltrate that spills into the epidermis with exocytosis. There are few eosinophils in the dermal infiltrate, and melanophages are evident.

Early Inflammatory Phase of Lichen Sclerosis et Atrophicus

Lichen sclerosis, particularly in its early inflammatory phase, can have histologic features mimicking MF [17, 19, 23]. Dense superficial dermal inflammatory cell infiltrate, sometimes in band-like fashion, usually occurs, and lymphocytic exocytosis in the epidermis could be quite prominent, which can be confusing with MF changes. However, the following histologic characteristics can be used quite reliably to differentiate from MF: edematous broadened upper dermis with homogenization above the inflammatory infiltrate and right beneath the epidermis, which becomes hyalinized with telangiectasia in late stage of the disease, and usually associated with epidermal atrophy and follicular plugging. Lack of lymphocytic atypia, haloed lymphocytes and Pautrier's microabscesses can further exclude MF.

Pityriasis Lichenoides Chronica

The papillary dermal lymphocytic infiltrate associated with epidermal lymphocyte exocytosis in biopsies of pityriasis lichenoides chronica (PLC) may raise consideration for the diagnosis of MF [24]. In PLC there are hyperkeratosis and parakeratosis, slight acanthosis, and often mild spongiosis in epidermis. Focal interface changes with basilar vacuolar degeneration and minimal exocytosis, sometimes associated with rare dyskeratotic keratinocytes, are present.

There is a relatively sparse superficial perivascular lymphohistiocytic infiltrate that can be accompanied by extravasated erythrocytes (Figure 5-10A and B). Long-lasting lesions may show papillary dermal fibroplasia. Few melanophages can also be present.

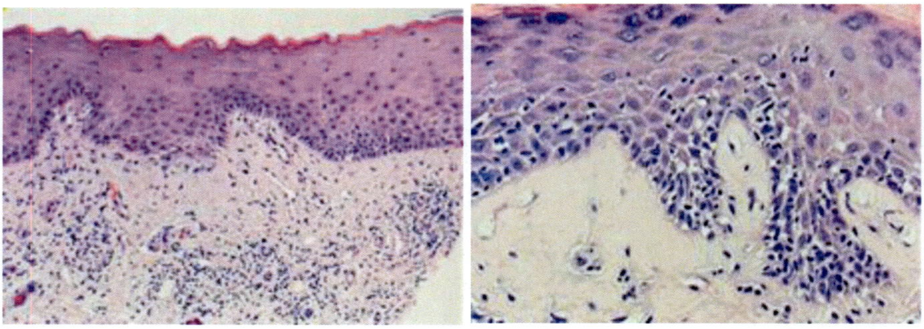

Figure 5-9. Lichen sclerosis et atrophicus. A (left): early inflammatory phase with moderately dense dermal lymphocytic infiltrate associated with early fibroplasia and discernible homogenization of the stroma. B (right): quite marked lymphocytic epidermal exocytosis, associated with moderate spongiosis and vacuolar interface changes. Prominent papillary dermal stromal hyalinization is evident.

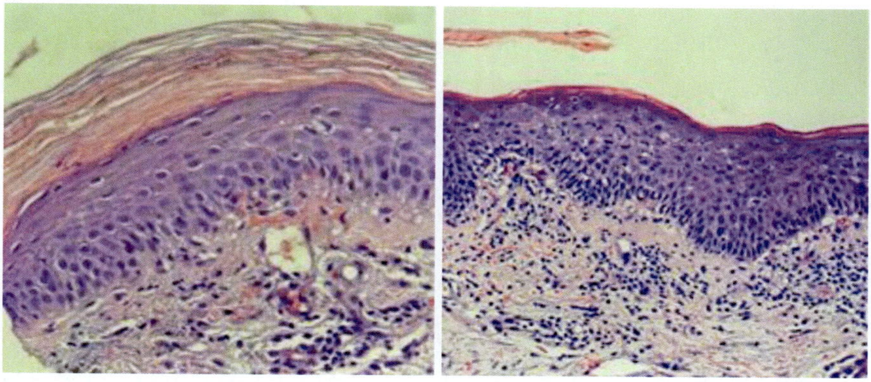

Figure 5-10. Pityriasis lichenoides chronica. A (left) and B (right): slight acanthosis with vacuolar interface changes and exocytosis of small lymphocytes in the epidermis, moderate dermal lymphocytic infiltrate associated with extravasated red blood cells.

Pigmented Purpuric Dermatoses

Pigmented purpuric dermatosis (PPD) includes a group of subtypes of related but different clinical entities with a similar histopathologic presentation. Although still debated, PPD has a component of lymphocytic vasculitis or capillaritis with vascular changes such as endothelial cell swelling, but usually no fibrin (Figure 5-11A). In the upper dermis, there is variable infiltrate of lymphocytes (predominantly CD4 positive T helper cells), histiocytes and CD1a positive dendritic cells. When the infiltrate is heavy, and sometimes in a lichenoid band-like pattern, such as in lichen aureus, and particularly coupled with conspicuous epidermal exocytosis of lymphocytes, PPD can present a diagnostic challenge in differentiating from MF. The presence of epidermal lymphocytes larger than dermal lymphocytes, atypia of dermal lymphocytes, and papillary dermal fibrosis favor a diagnosis of MF over PPD. On the other hand, extravasation of red blood cells, deposition of hemosiderin pigments, either in the form of hemosiderin-laden macrophages or lying freely in the superficial dermis, as well as focal interface/lichenoid changes with dyskeratotic keratinocytes would favor the diagnosis of PPD (Figure 5-11B and C). To complicate this matter further, there exists a condition called PPD/MF overlap [25], sometimes making a clear distinction between these two conditions very difficult or impossible. Therefore, careful clinical correlation with histologic evaluation, and ancillary investigation such as immunohistochemical stains and T cell gene rearrangement tests may be indicated [17]. Of note, cases of PPD with clonal T cell gene rearrangement have been reported, so the results of molecular testing should be interpreted within the context of the case as a whole.

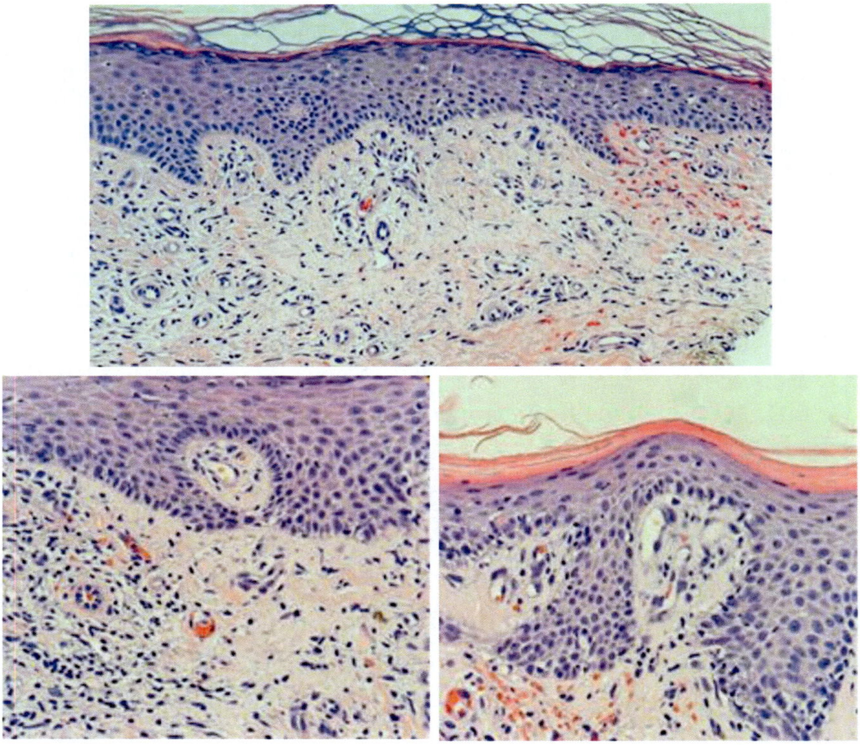

Figure 5-11. Pigmented purpuric dermatosis. A (top): moderate dermal lymphocytic infiltrate around prominent small vessels, and extravasation of red blood cells. B (bottom left): scattered hemosiderin pigment deposition in dermis. C (bottom right): vacuolar interface changes in the junction with occasional dyskeratotic keratinocytes.

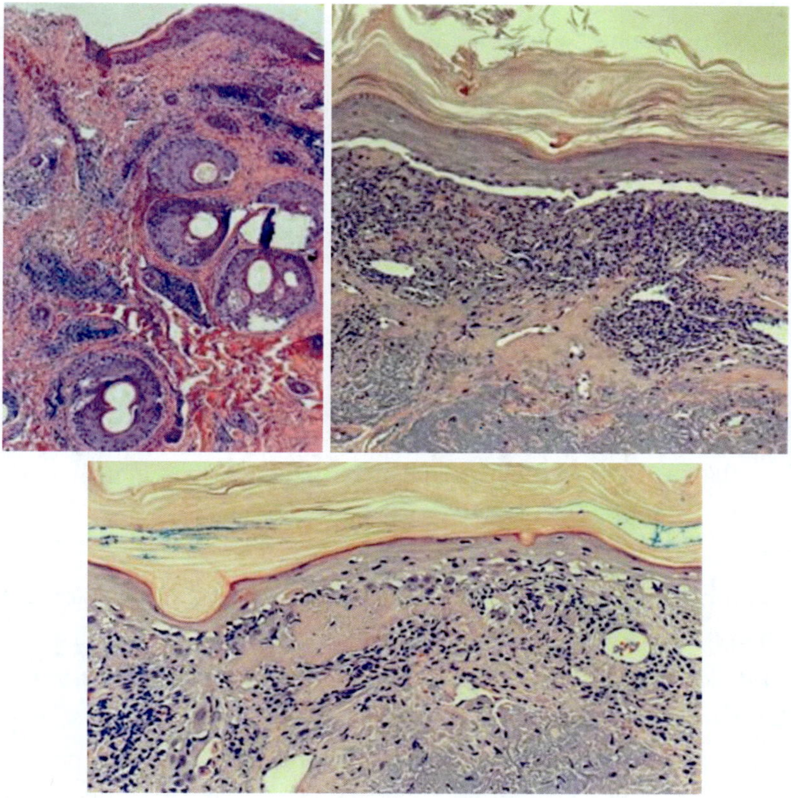

Figure 5-12. Discoid lupus erythematosis. A (top left): superficial and deep perivascular and periadnexal inflammatory infiltrate. B (top right): dense band-like lymphocytic infiltrate with cleft. C (bottom): prominent vacuolar interface changes with focal thickened basement membrane, lymphocytic exocytosis in the epidermis, and lymphocytic infiltrate in the superficial dermis.

Discoid Lupus Erythematosis

In most cases, the typical and characteristic histopathologic features of discoid lupus erythematodsis (DLE) can substantiate a definitive diagnosis fairly specifically. Rarely a dense superficial lymphocytic infiltrate, particularly in a band-like pattern, with "epidermotropism" of lymphocytes can simulate MF [26]. But in DLE, there is quite dense superficial and deep perivascular and periadnexal lymphocytic infiltrate (Figure 5-12A and B), sometimes with increased interstitial dermal mucin deposition. The epidermis is atrophic with basal layer vacuolar degeneration, associated with dyskeratotic keratinocytes. The basement membrane zone is thickened (Figure 5-12C). There is often keratin follicular plugging.

Psoriasiform Dermatitis

Psoriasis

Psoriasis has characteristic histopathologic features that usually would allow a fairly straightforward diagnosis, only rarely raising the concern of differentiation from MF when the superficial perivascular lymphocytic infiltrate is quite prominent, particularly associated with noticeable epidermal exocytosis of lymphocytes [27, 28].

In typical lesions, a psoriatic plaque will present confluent parakeratosis, with foci of neutrophils in the cornified layers, regular epidermal acanthosis with evenly elongated rete ridges with thinning of the suprapapillary plates, and attenuation of the granular layer, tortuous dilated capillaries in the papillary dermis approaching the lower surface of the epidermis, and a moderate lymphocytic perivascular inflammatory infiltrate that is usually not assuming the band-like pattern (Figure 5-13A and B). The constellation of the above mentioned unique histologic features is very helpful in separating psoriasis from MF, in the vast majority of cases, without any further work-up such as immunostains for T cell subpopulation and paired clonality testing needed.

Lichen Simplex Chronicus

Lichen simplex chronicus (LSC) per se rarely presents any opportunity for the necessity of differential diagnosis with MF, rather histologic changes of LSC can sometimes superimpose on lesions of MF. But occasionally one can see moderate superficial perivascular lymphocytic infiltrate, and even with slight exocytosis of epidermal haloed lymphocytes along the basal layer as shown in Figure 5-14.

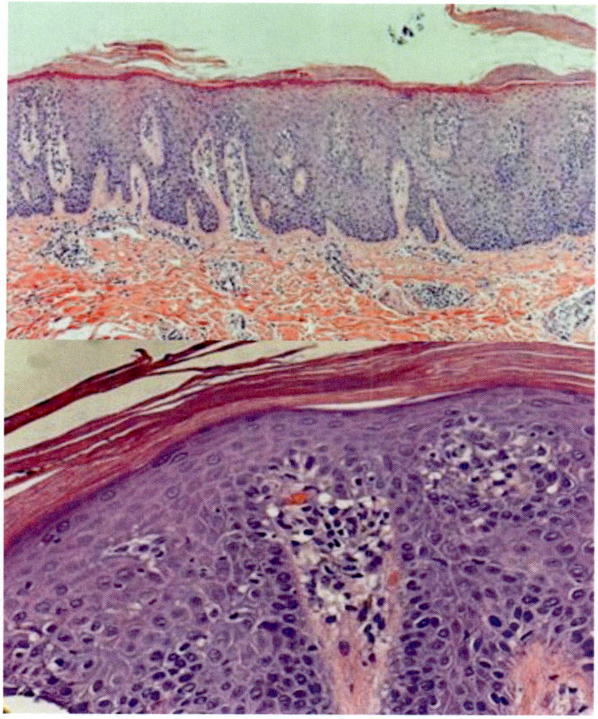

Figure 5-13. Psoriasis vulgaris. A (top): staggering and confluent parakeratosis overlying an epidermis with regular acanthosis, and a superficial perivascular inflammatory infiltrate. B (bottom): infiltrating lymphocytes in the papillary dermis and epidermis with certain degree of irregular nuclear contour.

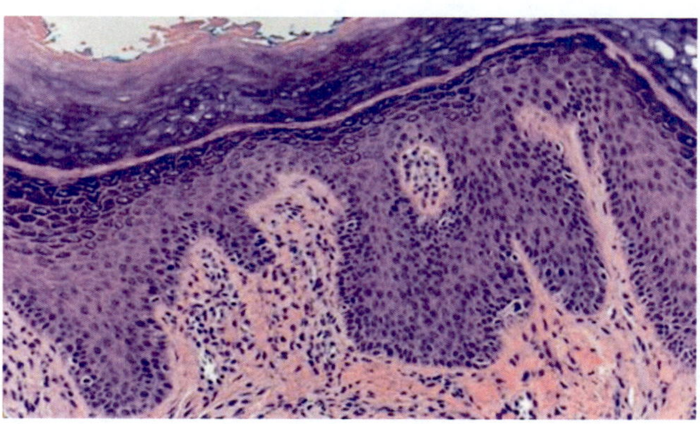

Figure 5-14. Lichen simplex chronicus. Irregular epidermal hyperplasia with focal hypergranulosis, and vertical fibrosis of the papillary dermis. There is lymphocytic infiltrate in the superficial dermis with scattered lymphocytes with halos along the basilar epidermis.

In LSC, a very thick layer of compact orthokeratosis resembling that seen on normal volar skin is usually present, overlying a hyperplastic epidermis with irregular acanthosis and prominent granular layer. A thickened papillary dermis is marked by fibrosis with bundles of collagen arranged in vertical streaks.

Secondary Syphilis

Syphilis is a great imitator clinically, and sometimes histopathologically as well. Considerable histopathologic variability in secondary syphilis can lead to misinterpretation and incorrect diagnosis. Nevertheless, the most frequent microscopic presentation of secondary syphilis can be summarized as following: psoriasiform epidermal hyperplasia with variable spongiosis and exocytosis of neutrophils and lymphocytes, vacuolar interface changes or lichenoid tissue reaction, superficial and deep perivascular and periadnexal mixed inflammatory infiltrate of lymphocytes and histiocytes, and usually associated with conspicuous plasma cells, vascular changes with angiogenesis and prominent endothelial cell swelling. At times when the dermal infiltrate becomes very dense and diffuse, a differential diagnosis of cutaneous lymphoma may warrant a further work-up in that direction, although the heterogeneous nature of the composition of the infiltrate is against the diagnosis of cutaneous lymphoproliferative disorders.

Occasionally, MF enters the differential diagnosis with secondary syphilis when the later presents with dense dermal infiltrate, particularly with band-like distribution, in association with conspicuous lymphocytic exocytosis in the epidermis [29, 30], even with single lymphocytes aligning along the basal layer (Figure 5-15A and B). Careful examination reveals plasma cells in the dermal infiltrate, which prompts immunohistochemical staining for the detection of Treponema pallidum. A positive result (Figure 5-15C) secures the correct diagnosis of secondary syphilis in this case.

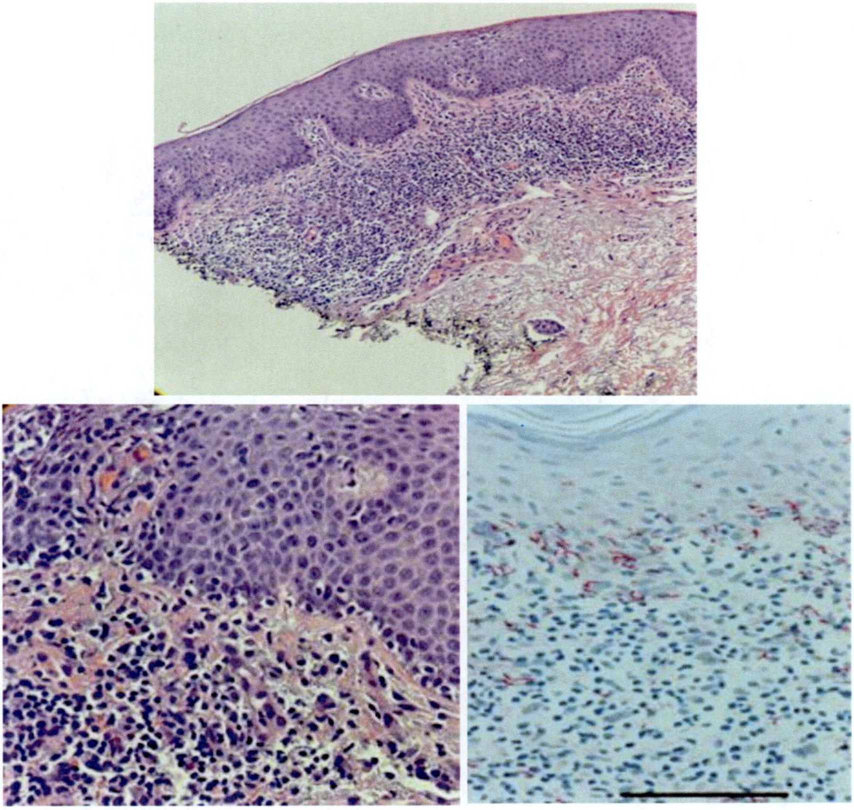

Figure 5-15. Secondary syphilis. A (top): dense band-like lymphocytic infiltrate in the papillary dermis. B (bottom left): lymphocytes with halos aligning along the basal layer of the epidermis, with papillary dermal lymphocytic infiltrate admixed with some plasma cells. C (bottom right): Immunostain positive for Treponema pallidum spirochetes.

I like to end this chapter with a rare and very unusual presentation of a secondary syphilis case to further illustrate the claim that syphilis is a great imitator, although this context is unrelated to the current chapter topic of histopathologic differential diagnosis of MF with benign inflammatory dermatoses.

At low power, there is very pronounced verrucous and pseudoepitheliomatous epidermal hyperplasia with dense mixed dermal inflammatory infiltrate. The infiltrate is composed of lymphocytes, neutrophils, histiocytes, few eosinophils, and very importantly, numerous plasma cells (Figure 5-16A and B).

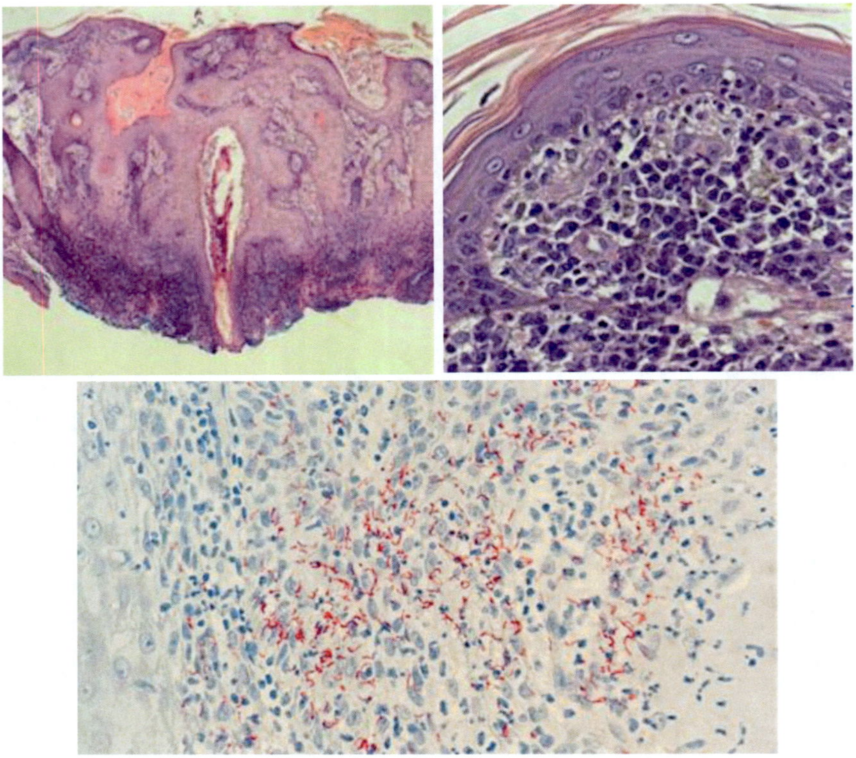

Figure 5-16. Secondary syphilis. A (top left): very prominent verrucous epidermal hyperplasia with dermal mixed inflammation. B (top right): numerous plasma cells in the dermal infiltrate. C (bottom): IHC for Treponema pallidum showing numerous spirochetes.

Although the clinical information accompanying this biopsy from the nose of a young female was to rule out sarcoidosis, the finding of numerous plasma cells triggered the ordering of immunohistochemical staining for detection of Treponema pallidum. As we can see in Figure 5-16C, numerous spirochetes are identified in the epidermis and dermis.

It is prudent to keep the diagnosis of syphilis in mind, particularly when one sees many plasma cells, and run the necessary additional staining for not missing an important diagnosis.

SUMMARY

Histopathologic diagnosis of patch and early plaque stage MF can be extremely difficult because almost all the histologic changes of early MF can variably occur in many benign inflammatory dermatoses. In this chapter the salient diagnostic histologic features of various benign dermatoses in three major categories of inflammatory tissue reaction pattern: spongiotic, interface/lichenoid, and psoriasiform, are discussed, particularly in correlation with differentiating from MF.

REFERENCES

[1] Cerroni, L., Mycosis fungoides-clinical and histopathologic features, differential diagnosis, and treatment. *Semin. Cutan. Med. Surg.,* 2018. 37(1): p. 2-10.

[2] Magro, C. M., M. C. Mihm, and A. N. Crowson, Mycosis fungoides, In: *The cutaneous lymphoid proliferations, A comprehensive textbook of lymphocytic infiltrates of the skin*, C. M. Magro, A. N. Crowson, and M. C. Mihm, Editors. 2007, Wiley-Liss. p. 267-299.

[3] Willemze, R., et al., WHO-EORTC classification for cutaneous lymphomas. *Blood*, 2005. 105(10): p. 3768-85.

[4] Zackheim, H. S. and T. H. McCalmont, Mycosis fungoides: the great imitator. *J. Am. Acad. Dermatol.*, 2002. 47(6): p. 914-8.

[5] Hodak, E. and I. Amitay-Laish, Mycosis fungoides: A great imitator. *Clin. Dermatol.*, 2019. 37(3): p. 255-267.

[6] Willemze, R., Mycosis fungoides variants-clinicopathologic features, differential diagnosis, and treatment. *Semin. Cutan. Med. Surg.*, 2018. 37(1): p. 11-17.

[7] Kelati, A., et al., Defining the mimics and clinico-histological diagnosis criteria for mycosis fungoides to minimize misdiagnosis. *Int. J. Womens Dermatol.*, 2017. 3(2): p. 100-106.

[8] Vandergriff, T., et al., Defining early mycosis fungoides: validation of a diagnostic algorithm proposed by the International Society for Cutaneous Lymphomas. *J. Cutan. Pathol.*, 2015. 42(5): p. 318-28.

[9] Ferrara, G., et al., Regarding the algorithm for the diagnosis of early mycosis fungoides proposed by the International Society for Cutaneous Lymphomas: suggestions from routine histopathology practice. *J. Cutan. Pathol.*, 2008. 35(6): p. 549-53.

[10] Jawed, S. I., et al., Primary cutaneous T-cell lymphoma (mycosis fungoides and Sézary syndrome): part I. Diagnosis: clinical and histopathologic features and new molecular and biologic markers. *J. Am. Acad. Dermatol.*, 2014. 70(2): p. 205 e1-16; quiz 221-2.

[11] Jawed, S. I., et al., Primary cutaneous T-cell lymphoma (mycosis fungoides and Sézary syndrome): part II. Prognosis, management, and future directions. *J. Am. Acad. Dermatol.,* 2014. 70(2): p. 223 e1-17; quiz 240-2.

[12] Raghavan, S. S. and J. Kim, Histopathologic approach to epidermotropic lymphocytic infiltrates. *Semin. Cutan. Med. Surg.*, 2018. 37(1): p. 56-60.

[13] Song, S. X., et al., Mycosis fungoides: report of the 2011 Society for Hematopathology/European Association for Haematopathology workshop. *Am. J. Clin. Pathol.*, 2013. 139(4): p. 466-90.

[14] Nickoloff, B. J., Light-microscopic assessment of 100 patients with patch/plaque-stage mycosis fungoides. *Am. J. Dermatopathol.*, 1988. 10(6): p. 469-77.

[15] Smoller, B. R., et al., Reassessment of histologic parameters in the diagnosis of mycosis fungoides. *Am. J. Surg. Pathol.*, 1995. 19(12): p. 1423-30.

[16] McKee, P. H., E. Calonie, and S. R. Granter, Chronic superficial dermatitis, In: *Pathology of the skin with clinical correlations*, P. H. McKee, E. Calonie, and S. R. Granter, Editors. 2005, Elsevier Mosby. p. 261-263.

[17] Reddy, K. and J. Bhawan, Histologic mimickers of mycosis fungoides: a review. *J. Cutan. Pathol.*, 2007. 34(7): p. 519-25.

[18] Shamim, H., et al., Mycosis fungoides with spongiosis: A potential diagnostic pitfall. *J. Cutan. Pathol.*, 2019. 46(9): p. 645-652.

[19] Arps, D. P., et al., Selected inflammatory imitators of mycosis fungoides: histologic features and utility of ancillary studies. *Arch. Pathol. Lab. Med.,* 2014. 138(10): p. 1319-27.

[20] Rao, B. K., J. Merino, and I. Rahman Mycosis Fungoides Mimicking Lichen Planus. *Journal of Cutaneous Pathology*, 2008. 32.

[21] Gorouhi, F., P. Davari, and N. Fazel, Cutaneous and mucosal lichen planus: a comprehensive review of clinical subtypes, risk factors, diagnosis, and prognosis. *Scientific World Journal*, 2014. 2014: p. 742826.

[22] Al-Hoqail, I. A. and R. I. Crawford, Benign lichenoid keratoses with histologic features of mycosis fungoides: clinicopathologic description of a clinically significant histologic pattern. *J. Cutan. Pathol.*, 2002. 29(5): p. 291-4.

[23] Citarella, L., et al., Lichen sclerosus with histopathologic features simulating early mycosis fungoides. *Am. J. Dermatopathol.*, 2003. 25(6): p. 463-5.

[24] Borra, T., et al., Pityriasis Lichenoides, Atypical Pityriasis Lichenoides, and Related Conditions: A Study of 66 Cases. *Am. J. Surg. Pathol.,* 2018. 42(8): p. 1101-1112.

[25] Toro, J. R., C. A. Sander, and P. E. LeBoit, Persistent pigmented purpuric dermatitis and mycosis fungoides: simulant, precursor, or both? A study by light microscopy and molecular methods. *Am. J. Dermatopathol.*, 1997. 19(2): p. 108-18.

[26] Friss, A. B., et al., Chronic cutaneous lupus erythematosus mimicking mycosis fungoides. *J. Am. Acad. Dermatol.*, 1995. 33(5 Pt 2): p. 891-5.

[27] Azizpour, A., et al., Psoriasiform mycosis fungoides: a rare form of the disease with review of the literature. *Dermatol. Online J.,* 2017. 23(9).

[28] Doukaki, S., M. Arico, and M. R. Bongiorno, A Rare Presentation of Mycosis Fungoides Mimicking Psoriasis Vulgaris. *Case Rep. Dermatol.*, 2009. 1(1): p. 60-65.

[29] Levin, D. L., et al., Secondary syphilis mimicking mycosis fungoides. *J. Am. Acad. Dermatol.*, 1980. 3(1): p. 92-4.

[30] Flamm, A., et al., Histopathologic features distinguishing secondary syphilis from its mimickers. *J. Am. Acad. Dermatol.*, 2020. 82(1): p. 156-160.

In: Mycosis Fungoides and Sézary Syndrome ISBN: 978-1-68507-093-9
Editors: X. Zhang and L. Sokol

Chapter 6

CLINICAL VARIANTS OF MYCOSIS FUNGOIDES

Sarah Moore, MD, and James Isom*, MD
Department of Dermatology and Cutaneous Surgery,
University of South Florida Morsani College of Medicine,
Tampa, FL, US

INTRODUCTION

Mycosis fungoides (MF) is protean in its presentation, and therefore, numerous variants of mycosis fungoides have been reported in the literature (see Table 6-1) [1]. The variants can be broadly divided into clinical variants, histopathologic variants, and phenotypic variants [2]. Among clinical variants, a subset demonstrates unique histopathologic findings. The World Health Organization (WHO) and European Organization for Research and Treatment of Cancer (EORTC) provided an updated consensus classification for primary cutaneous lymphomas in 2018, and they (WHO-EORTC) now formally recognize the following mycosis fungoides variants:

* Corresponding Author's Email: jamesisommd@gmail.com.

folliculotropic mycosis fungoides, pagetoid reticulosis, and granulomatous slack skin [3]. The formally recognized and most commonly reported clinical variants are discussed below.

Table 6-1. Clinical variants of mycosis fungoides

Clinical variants with "conventional" histopathological features	Clinical variants with peculiar histopathological features
Acanthosis nigricans-like mycosis fungoides Atopic dermatitis-like mycosis fungoides Erythrodermic mycosis fungoides* Hypopigmented mycosis fungoides* Icthyosiform mycosis fungoides Palmoplantar mycosis fungoides Papular mycosis fungoides Papuloerythroderma of Ofuji (subset of cases) Parapsoriasis ("large patch") Perioral dermatitis-like mycosis fungoides Pityriasis lichenoides-like mycosis fungoides (clinical variant) Psoriasiform mycosis fungoides Unilesional (solitary) mycosis fungoides Zosteriform mycosis fungoides	Adnexotropic mycosis fungoides, including: Pilotropic (folliculotropic) mycosis fungoides*, mycosis fungoides with eruptive infundibular cysts and comedones, and syringotropic mycosis fungoides Anetodermic mycosis fungoides Bullous (vesiculobullous) mycosis fungoides Dyshidrotic mycosis fungoides Epidermal mucinosis in mycosis fungoides Granulomatous slack skin* Hyperpigmented mycosis fungoides* "Invisible" mycosis fungoides Pagetoid reticulosis (Worringer-Kolopp type)* Poikilodermatous mycosis fungoides* Purpuric mycosis fungoides Pustular mycosis fungoides Verrucous/hyperkeratotic mycosis fungoides

Adapted and modified from Cerroni [2].
*Discussed below.

Folliculotropic Mycosis Fungoides

Folliculotropic MF (FMF) is the most common clinical variant of MF recognized by the WHO-EORTC classification system, accounting for 10% of all MF cases [4, 5]. FMF is distinguished from classic MF by the presence of folliculotropic lymphocytic infiltrate, often with mucinous degeneration of follicular epithelium (follicular mucinosis), with a tendency to affect the skin on the head and neck. Follicular infiltration by neoplastic T cells is not unique to FMF and can also be seen in folliculocentric lymphomatoid papulosis, CD8+ aggressive epidermotropic cytotoxic CTCL, and classic MF. Characterization of FMF requires clinicopathologic correlation [6, 7].

Clinical Presentation

FMF preferentially affects the skin of the head and neck region and is classically characterized by grouped follicular papules, often with concurrent alopecia. Clinical presentation can be variable, with some patients presenting with acneiform lesions (Fig. 6-1); follicle-centered patches, plaques, or tumors; and keratosis pilaris-like eruption on trunk and extremities [4, 8-12]. Rare cases have been reported of FMF presenting as a solitary lesion or erythroderma [13, 14]. One highly characteristic and common finding is infiltrated plaques and alopecia affecting the eyebrows. Clinically, patients often endorse severe pruritus, which can be used as a reliable measure of disease activity [15].

FMF more commonly affects adults, predominantly affecting males; however, children and adolescents can also be affected [4, 8-11, 16]. Children typically present with hypopigmented folliclocentric patches associated with alopecia [12]. Children and adolescents are also more frequently affected by alopecia mucinosa, which has an excellent prognosis [17]. This idiopathic and benign form of follicular mucinosis presents with singular or a few patches of alopecia with follicular accentuation. The relationship between alopecia mucinosa and FMF is still debated [18].

Generally, if lesions are more widespread and persistent, then the diagnosis of FMF is favored.

Histopathology

FMF is characterized by folliculotropic infiltrates of atypical neoplastic T cells, with variable, but typically absent, involvement of the interfollicular epidermis. Many cases are associated with mucinous degeneration of the hair follicle (follicular mucinosis). The absence of follicular mucinosis in the setting of folliculotropic infiltrates is often referred to as pilotropic MF [19]. Infiltration of eccrine glands (syringotropism) can also be present and is often reported as adnexotropic MF/syringotropic MF [20, 21].

Early stage FMF is characterized clinically as follicle-centered patches, keratosis pilaris-like and acniform lesions. Histologically, these lesions have sparse perifollicular infiltrates, with variable amounts of reactive T cells, histiocytes, and rarely eosinophils. Advanced stage FMF, clinically presenting as nodules, tumors, or erythroderma, has a more robust dermal infiltrate including increased blast cells and eosinophils.

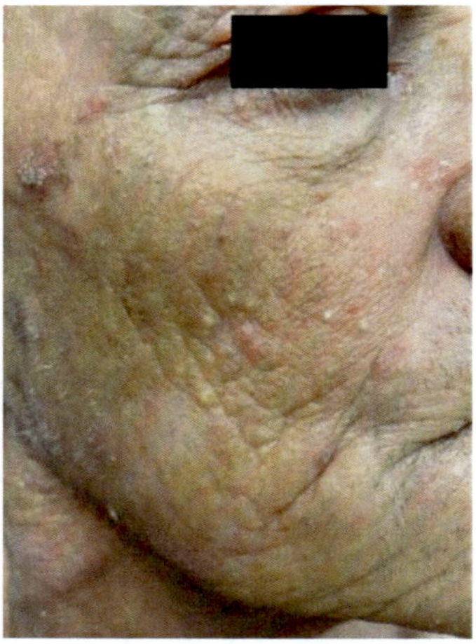

Figure 6-1. Acneiform lesions in a patient with folliculotropic mycosis fungoides.

Neoplastic cells for FMF are small- to medium-sized, or less frequently large, T cells with hyperchromatic cerebriform nuclei. These cells almost always stain CD3+/CD4+/CD8- [20]. Colloidal iron or Alcian blue stains can be helpful to identify follicular mucinosis. A majority of cases have clonal T-cell gene rearrangement. Some cases may have a small population of CD30+ blast cells or CD20+ B cells [20]. The presence of blast cells exceeding 25% or clusters of blast cells is defined as large-cell transformation and is seen in more than 20% of FMF cases [8, 10, 11].

Prognosis and Treatment

Classically, FMF has been considered a more aggressive clinical phenotype of MF, behaving similarly to tumor-stage MF [4, 8, 10]. According to a large cutaneous lymphoma registry, the 5-year disease specific survival of FMF is 75% [3]. More recent clinicopathologic studies describe a subgroup of FMF patients whose clinical course is more analogous to early-stage classic MF. This subgroup of patients has an excellent prognosis, with 5- and 10-year disease specific survival comparable to early patch stage MF [11, 12, 22]. Factors leading to increased mortality include age, advanced stage, large-cell transformation, and secondary bacterial infections [10, 11].

Distinguishing between indolent and aggressive subgroups of FMF is important when determining appropriate treatments. Some histopathologic features that can be helpful in distinguishing the more aggressive subgroup include percentage of atypical cells, percentage of Ki-67 positive cells, size of neoplastic T cells, percentage of blast cells, and presence of interfollicular epidermotropism [23].

A stepwise approach to treatment is often preferred [11]. Early-stage or indolent FMF can be treated with skin-directed therapies, including topical steroids, topical nitrogen mustard, or psoralen plus ultraviolet A (PUVA). For more aggressive FMF, the deeper infiltrate of atypical T cells in the hair follicle renders skin-directed therapy minimally effective. These patients are treated with PUVA combined with interferon alfa and/or oral retinoids; local radiotherapy alone or in combination with PUVA; or total skin electron beam irradiation [8, 10].

Pagetoid Reticulosis

Pagetoid reticulosis (PR) is a rare clinical variant of MF, characterized by a solitary patch or plaque with pagetoid infiltrate of neoplastic T cells [15].

Clinical Presentation

PR typically presents as a slowly progressive, solitary, psoriasiform hyperkeratotic plaque or patch localized to the extremities, most commonly affecting acral skin. A disseminated version has been reported known as Ketron-Goodman type, but the term PR exclusively refers to the localized form (Woringer-Kolopp type) [24, 25]. Any age group can be affected by PR.

Histopathology

PR is characterized by prominent epidermotropism of small- to medium-sized atypical T lymphocytes. The epidermis exhibits acanthosis and hyperkeratosis. The numerous pagetoid cells give the epidermis a buck-shot appearance. The neoplastic lymphocytes have cerebriform nuclei with abundant, vacuolated cytoplasm. Neoplastic lymphocytes are almost exclusively found in the epidermis, although the superficial dermis can have an inflammatory infiltrate of small lymphocytes. Eosinophils are generally absent [26].

Immunohistochemistry of neoplastic T cells can be variable, expressing CD3+/CD4+/CD8-, CD3+/CD4-/CD8+, or CD3+/CD4-/CD8- cells. CD7 is generally negative, while CD30+ cells are present in a majority of cases [20].

The neoplastic T cells are generall α/β T cells, rarely γ/δ T cells [26]. Ki-67 proliferative index is usually high.

Prognosis and Treatment

PR typically follows an indolent course. Patients have an excellent prognosis with 5-year disease specific survival of 100% [3]. Extracutaneous disease progression has never been reported. Involved skin is localized and well-circumscribed, making local radiotherapy or surgical excision the treatment of choice [26]. PR can also be treated with a variety of skin-directed therapies including topical steroids, topical nitrogen mustard, PUVA, narrowband ultraviolet B (NB-UVB), and imiquimod.

Granulomatous Slack Skin

Granulomatous slack skin (GSS) is a rare variant of MF and accounts for less than 1% of MF cases [3].

Clinical Presentation

Initially, GSS presents similarly to patch or plaque stage classic MF, with erythematous to violaceous patches or plaques with atrophic surface [27, 28]. Over the course of years, the plaques slowly expand creating redundant, pendulous skin folds. Intertriginous areas are favored, with axilla and inguinal region being most common [28, 29]. GSS is generally asymptomatic, but plaques may ulcerate [27]. GSS can affect any age or gender, although it preferentially affects middle-aged men [29, 30].

Extracutaneous manifestations, including lymph node involvement, are less common in GSS when compared to other types of MF, although infiltration into the bronchial mucosa may be seen [27, 31]. Despite the indolent course of GSS, one-third to half of patients will develop another lymphoproliferative disorder [29, 32].

Histopathology

Histologically, GSS exhibits variable infiltrate of small- to medium-sized monoclonal T cells intermixed with scattered multinucleated giant cells and macrophages [27]. Mixed inflammatory infiltrate with eosinophils, histocytes, and plasma cells is typically seen [28]. The lymphocytic infiltrate can be perivascular or diffuse throughout the dermis and is typically CD3+/CD4+/CD8-/CD45RO+ [28]. TCR gene rearrangement is common [28, 33]. Epidermal involvement is variable with some cases showing significant epidermotropism and some with complete lack of lymphocytes in the epidermis [28, 34].

GSS also shows loss of elastic fibers through elastophagocytosis and consumption of lymphocytes by multinucleated giant cells (emperipolesis). This elastic fiber loss can be demonstrated using an orcein stain [34]. One characteristic finding in GSS is multinucleated giant cells with more than 10 nuclei, although this feature can also be seen in granulomatous MF. Granulomatous MF is the primary histologic differential for GSS, as they both contain granulomatous infiltrate with CD4+ clonal T cells, multinucleated giant cells, and loss of elastic tissue [28]. With these similarities, clinical correlation is required to differentiate between GSS and granulomatous MF as they have different clinical presentations and prognosis. Skin redundancy in flexural areas helps distinguish GSS.

Prognosis and Treatment

GSS has an indolent course with 5-year disease specific survival of 100% [3]. Although GSS is not life-threatening, the risk for poor outcomes is determined by the development of concomitant lymphoproliferative disorders. The most common associated diseases include Hodgkin lymphoma, non-Hodgkin lymphoma, acute myeloid leukemia, classic MF, among others [28, 32, 35]. Development of these lymphoproliferative disorders has been reported in as high as 50% of cases [32]. It is important to make the clinical distinction between GSS and granulomatous MF, as granulomatous MF only has a 5-year disease specific survival of 66% [33, 36].

Treatment of GSS is largely unsuccessful. The disease typically follows a slowly progressive clinical course with limited response to treatment. Even surgical excision often is followed by recurrence [28, 30, 32, 37]. Other treatment options include PUVA, radiotherapy, chemotherapy, corticosteroids, interferon, nitrogen mustard, among other common treatments for MF [27, 29]. Partial remission has been reported with the use of PUVA or carmustine [28]. Despite the unsatisfactory treatment results, these patients need to be followed closely to monitor for the development of secondary lymphoproliferative disorders.

Hypopigmented Mycosis Fungoides

Hypopigmented MF is a variant that was first reported in the 1970's [38, 39] with case series appearing in the ensuing decade [40, 41]. Hypopigmented MF constitutes approximately 20% of MF cases according to two studies [42, 43]. Hypopigmented MF is the most common subtype in pediatric patients, and among adult patients, age of onset is lower [42]. In addition, it is the most common subtype in patients with skin of color [44].

Clinical Presentation

Hypopigmented MF lesions are found on the trunk, buttocks, and proximal extremities. The face, hands, and feet are typically spared. The hypopigmented lesions present with variable sizes ranging from macules to patches and variable morphology, including round-to-oval shaped lesions as well as irregular streaks [44]. Patients often endorse pruritus but deny systemic symptoms. The variable presentation yields a large differential (e.g., pityriasis versicolor, pityriasis alba, and vitiligo) and can delay diagnosis [42, 44].

Histopathology

Histology demonstrates similar findings to classic MF. Notably, Fontana-Masson studies demonstrate that epidermal melanin is not significantly decreased, and Melan-A immunohistochemical studies highlight preserved melanocytes at the dermal-epidermal junction - in contrast to vitiligo. The neoplastic lymphocytes tend to be cytotoxic T cell (CD8+), although helper T cell (CD4+) immunophenotype has been observed [44]. Ultrastructural studies demonstrate spherical, incompletely melanized melanosomes, which are not specific for hypopigmented MF but may explain the peculiar clinical and histologic findings [40].

Prognosis and Treatment

Hypopigmented MF has a favorable prognosis and rarely progresses past stage IB [42]. Topical therapy and phototherapy are the first-line treatments. As observed in classic MF, phototherapy has an excellent response rate in hypopigmented MF. In addition, the hypopigmented lesions often repigment after treatment [42, 45].

Hyperpigmented Mycosis Fungoides

Hyperpigmented MF is an uncommon variant that interestingly also favors patients with a darker complexion. One study reports 87.5% of patients in their case series as having Fitzpatrick IV skin type [46]. Although pigmentary changes are seen in regressing MF lesions, hyperpigmented MF presents with pigment alteration prior to therapy - a key distinction [47].

Clinical Presentation

Hyperpigmented MF presents as hyperpigmented patches and/or plaques, which can be asymptomatic or pruritic. The lesions are variably well-defined, and the morphologic spectrum spans from well-defined, distinct patches to ill-defined involvement of large areas of skin. Uncommonly, patients are initially diagnosed with post-inflammatory pigment alteration (PIPA). Typically, hyperpigmented lesions are the sole manifestation of MF, but hypopigmented, ichthyosiform, or poikilodermatous lesions can coexist. Classic erythematous lesions have not been observed in patients with hyperpigmented MF [46, 47].

Histopathology

Histology reveals the classic MF findings of epidermotropism, Pautrier abscess formation, and atypical lymphocytes. In addition, hyperpigmented MF demonstrates interface changes and variable melanophages. Necrotic keratinocytes within the epidermis are not uncommon [46, 47].

The immunophenotype is more commonly cytotoxic T cell (CD8+) than helper T cell (CD4+). The proclivity for a CD8+ immunoprofile may be responsible for the interface change and resulting pigment incontinence, although most cases of MF with a cytotoxic immunophenotype do not demonstrate hyperpigmentation. Patients with variable lesion morphology do not also exhibit variable immunophenotypes [46].

Prognosis and Treatment

Hyperpigmened MF typically follows an indolent course, behaving similarly to early-stage classic MF. This variant needs to be distinguished from classic MF with CD8+ phenotype, which typically has a more aggressive course [46, 48]. Treatment is based on stage and is similar to classic MF. Options include PUVA, topical steroids, oral retinoids, topical chemotherapy, or interferon [48]. Using combination therapy has become increasingly popular.

Erythrodermic Mycosis Fungoides

Eythrodermic MF is defined as MF with erythroderma caused by coalescing lesions and without blood involvement [49, 50]. Although some consider Sézary syndrome and erythrodermic MF to be part of an erythrodermic cutaneous lymphoma spectrum, the putative progenitor T cells arise from different subsets [51]. Therefore, the erythrodermic MF and Sézary syndrome should be considered distinct entities despite their similarities in clinical appearance.

Clinical Presentation

Patient demographics are the same as in classic MF with the prototypical patient being an older white man. Patients present with erythroderma (i.e., erythema and edema effecting >90% of skin surface area) (Fig. 6-2). The severity can vary from mild erythema to exfoliative erythema with keratoderma and fissures of acral surfaces. Secondary to skin changes, patients suffer from hypothermia, electrolyte imbalances, and hair loss [52].

Histopathology

Erythrodermic MF is histologically identical to classic MF, and the immunoprofile is also the same as classic MF (CD3+/CD4+/CD8- with aberrant loss of CD5 and/or CD7). Sézary syndrome can exhibit similar findings. Importantly, peripheral blood flow cytometry studies do not detect circulating neoplastic T cells - as seen in Sézary syndrome [53].

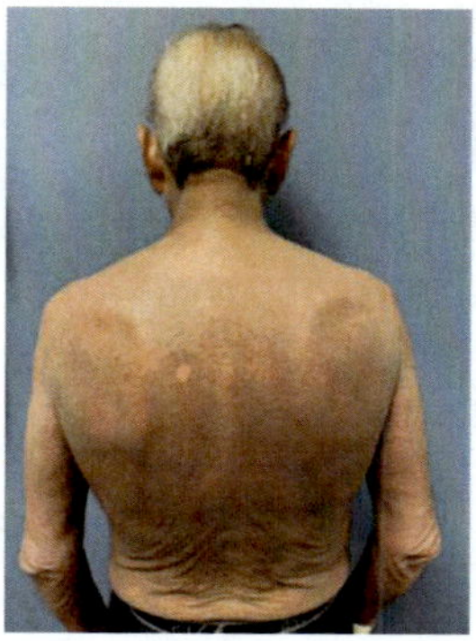

Figure 6-2. A patient with erythrodermic mycosis fungoides.

Prognosis and Treatment

The significant overlap between erythrodermic MF and Sézary syndrome makes distinction difficult. As a result, prognosis and therapy response are unclear. Historically, the prognosis of erythrodermic MF has been considered poor with median overall survival reported as low as 5.0 years [54]. However, a recent study reported more favorable outcomes in patients with clearly defined erythrodermic MF [52]. Extracorporeal photopheresis, total skin electron beam therapy, and phototherapy as well as systemic medications (specifically, alemtuzumab) are the mainstays of therapy. The diffuse cutaneous involvement of disease typically precludes topical medications.

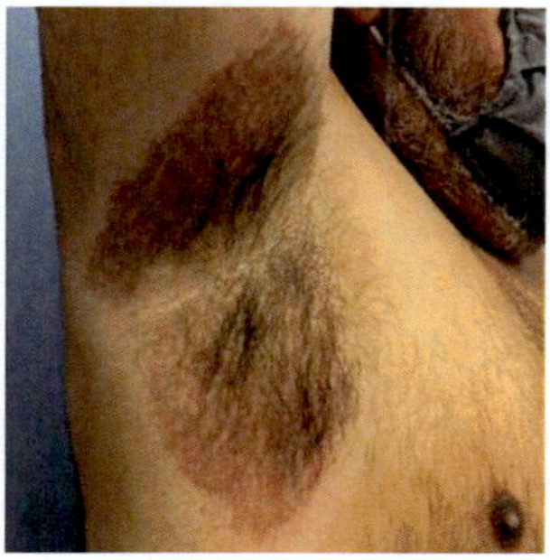

Figure 6-3. Poikilodermatous axillary lesion in a patient with poikilodermatous mycosis fungoides.

Poikilodermatous Mycosis Fungoides

Poikilodermatous MF was originally described as “poikiloderma atrophicans vasculare” by Jacobi in 1908, and eventually, it was classified as a subtype of MF by Samman in 1972 [55]. Officially, the WHO-EORTC classification does not recognize poikilodermatous MF as a subtype despite its long history and rather unique features [3]. Classically, the lesions are characterized as atrophic macules and patches with admixed hyper- and hypo-pigmentation and telangiectasias (Fig. 6-3).

Clinical Presentation

Patients with poikilodermatous MF typically present at a slightly younger age with a median age at diagnosis of 44 years. Also, the duration from clinical symptom onset to diagnosis was slightly longer in patients with poikilodermatous MF than classic MF (10 years vs 6-7 years) [55]. The lesions favor the breasts and buttocks although they can be widespread [2]. Dermoscopy of poikilodermatous MF lesions reveals pale areas, studded with fine red dots or hairpin vessels and intervening septa of pigmented dots [56].

Histopathology

Poikilodermatous MF is typically CD4+/CD8- with variable loss of pan-T-cell antigens (e.g., CD2, CD5, CD7, etc.). However, CD4-/CD8+ poikilodermatous can occur (38% of cases in one study), and it is more common than CD8+ classic MF [55]. Rarely, a cytotoxic immunophenotype (CD56+/TIA+) can occur within the setting of an either CD4+/CD8- profile or CD4-/CD8+ profile. Poikilodermatous MF with a cytotoxic immunophenotype must be distinguished via clinicopathologic correlation from more aggressive lymphomas such as primary cutaneous aggressive epidermotropic CD8+ cytotoxic T cell lymphoma, primary cutaneous gamma/delta T cell lymphoma, and extranodal NK/T cell lymphoma (nasal type) [57, 58].

Prognosis and Treatment

The prognosis for poikilodermatous MF is slightly better than classic MF. Specifically, poikilodermatous MF has a lower risk for disease progression and a higher disesase-specific survival than classic MF [5, 59]. Patients typically respond well to phototherapy, and it has the best response rate in patients with poikilodermatous MF [55].

Conclusion

The WHO-EORTC officially recognizes that MF variants are the most essential for prognosis and treatment, and fortunately, they are the most well-studied. A complete discussion of all variants is beyond the scope of this chapter. Cerroni's Skin Lymphoma: The Illustrated Guide [2] provides one of the most complete guides to treatments of cutaneous lymphoma in general and mycosis fungoides in particular. Still, new variants are bound to appear in the literature, and therefore, primary sources should not be neglected when encountering an unusual clinical presentation suspicious for mycosis fungoides.

References

[1] Kazakov, D. V., G. Burg, and W. Kempf, Clinicopathological spectrum of mycosis fungoides. *J Eur Acad Dermatol Venereol*, 2004. 18(4): p. 397-415.

[2] Cerroni, L., *Skin lymphoma: the illustrated guide.* 2020, John Wiley & Sons: Hoboken, NJ. p. 1 online resource.

[3] Willemze, R., et al., The 2018 update of the WHO-EORTC classification for primary cutaneous lymphomas. *Blood*, 2019. 133(16): p. 1703-1714.

[4] van Doorn, R., E. Scheffer, and R. Willemze, Follicular mycosis fungoides, a distinct disease entity with or without associated follicular mucinosis: a clinicopathologic and follow-up study of 51 patients. *Arch Dermatol*, 2002. 138(2): p. 191-8.

[5] Agar, N. S., et al., Survival outcomes and prognostic factors in mycosis fungoides/Sézary syndrome: validation of the revised International Society for Cutaneous Lymphomas/European Organisation for Research and Treatment of Cancer staging proposal. *J Clin Oncol*, 2010. 28(31): p. 4730-9.

[6] Kempf, W., et al., Follicular lymphomatoid papulosis revisited: a study of 11 cases, with new histopathological findings. *J Am Acad Dermatol*, 2013. 68(5): p. 809-16.

[7] Robson, A., et al., Aggressive epidermotropic cutaneous CD8+ lymphoma: a cutaneous lymphoma with distinct clinical and pathological features. Report of an EORTC Cutaneous Lymphoma Task Force Workshop. *Histopathology*, 2015. 67(4): p. 425-41.

[8] Gerami, P., et al., Folliculotropic mycosis fungoides: an aggressive variant of cutaneous T-cell lymphoma. *Arch Dermatol*, 2008. 144(6): p. 738-46.

[9] Lehman, J. S., et al., Folliculotropic mycosis fungoides: single-center study and systematic review. *Arch Dermatol*, 2010. 146(6): p. 607-13.

[10] Wieser, I., et al., Clinical characteristics, risk factors and long-term outcome of 114 patients with folliculotropic mycosis fungoides. *Arch Dermatol Res*, 2017. 309(6): p. 453-459.

[11] van Santen, S., et al., Clinical Staging and Prognostic Factors in Folliculotropic Mycosis Fungoides. *JAMA Dermatol*, 2016. 152(9): p. 992-1000.

[12] Hodak, E., et al., New insights into folliculotropic mycosis fungoides (FMF): A single-center experience. *J Am Acad Dermatol*, 2016. 75(2): p. 347-55.

[13] Kempf, W., et al., Unilesional follicular mycosis fungoides: report of two cases with progression to tumor stage and review of the literature. *J Cutan Pathol*, 2012. 39(9): p. 853-60.

[14] Amitay-Laish, I., et al., Unilesional folliculotropic mycosis fungoides: a unique variant of cutaneous lymphoma. *J Eur Acad Dermatol Venereol*, 2016. 30(1): p. 25-9.

[15] Willemze, R., Mycosis fungoides variants-clinicopathologic features, differential diagnosis, and treatment. *Semin Cutan Med Surg*, 2018. 37(1): p. 11-17.

[16] Boulos, S., et al., Clinical presentation, immunopathology, and treatment of juvenile-onset mycosis fungoides: a case series of 34 patients. *J Am Acad Dermatol*, 2014. 71(6): p. 1117-26.

[17] Alikhan, A., et al., Pediatric follicular mucinosis: presentation, histopathology, molecular genetics, treatment, and outcomes over an 11-year period at the Mayo Clinic. *Pediatr Dermatol*, 2013. 30(2): p. 192-8.

[18] Cerroni, L., et al., Follicular mucinosis: a critical reappraisal of clinicopathologic features and association with mycosis fungoides and Sézary syndrome. *Arch Dermatol*, 2002. 138(2): p. 182-9.

[19] Vergier, B., et al., Pilotropic cutaneous T-cell lymphoma without mucinosis. A variant of mycosis fungoides? French Study Group of Cutaneous Lymphomas. *Arch Dermatol*, 1996. 132(6): p. 683-7.

[20] Gerami, P. and J. Guitart, The spectrum of histopathologic and immunohistochemical findings in folliculotropic mycosis fungoides. *Am J Surg Pathol*, 2007. 31(9): p. 1430-8.

[21] de Masson, A., et al., Syringotropic mycosis fungoides: clinical and histologic features, response to treatment, and outcome in 19 patients. *J Am Acad Dermatol*, 2014. 71(5): p. 926-34.

[22] Tomasini, C., et al., Spiky follicular mycosis fungoides: a clinicopathologic study of 8 cases. *J Cutan Pathol*, 2015. 42(3): p. 164-72.

[23] van Santen, S., et al., Plaque stage folliculotropic mycosis fungoides: histopathologic features and prognostic factors in a series of 40 patients. *J Cutan Pathol*, 2020. 47(3): p. 241-250.

[24] Willemze, R., et al., WHO-EORTC classification for cutaneous lymphomas. *Blood*, 2005. 105(10): p. 3768-85.

[25] Haghighi, B., et al., Pagetoid reticulosis (Woringer-Kolopp disease): an immunophenotypic, molecular, and clinicopathologic study. *Mod Pathol*, 2000. 13(5): p. 502-10.

[26] Virmani, P., P. L. Myskowski, and M. Pulitzer, Unusual variants of mycosis fungoides. *Diagn Histopathol* (Oxf), 2016. 22(4): p. 142-151.

[27] Goldsztajn, K. O., et al., Granulomatous slack skin. Histopathology diagnosis preceding clinical manifestations by 12 years. *J Dermatol Case Rep*, 2012. 6(4): p. 108-12.

[28] Kempf, W., et al., Granulomatous mycosis fungoides and granulomatous slack skin: a multicenter study of the Cutaneous Lymphoma Histopathology Task Force Group of the European Organization for Research and Treatment of Cancer (EORTC). *Arch Dermatol*, 2008. 144(12): p. 1609-17.

[29] van Haselen, C. W., et al., Granulomatous slack skin. Report of three patients with an updated review of the literature. *Dermatology,* 1998. 196(4): p. 382-91.

[30] Balus, L., F. Bassetti, and G. Gentili, Granulomatous slack skin. *Arch Dermatol*, 1985. 121(2): p. 250-2.

[31] van Doorn, R., et al., Mycosis fungoides: disease evolution and prognosis of 309 Dutch patients. *Arch Dermatol,* 2000. 136(4): p. 504-10.

[32] Noto, G., et al., Granulomatous slack skin: report of a case associated with Hodgkin's disease and a review of the literature. *Br J Dermatol*, 1994. 131(2): p. 275-9.

[33] Sheng, Y., et al., Granulomatous slack skin: assessment of disease progression and treatment response using positron emission tomography/computed tomography. *Clin Lymphoma Myeloma*, 2009. 9(6): p. 455-8.

[34] Tsang, W. Y., et al., Granulomatous slack skin. *Histopathology*, 1994. 25(1): p. 49-55.

[35] Miyagaki, T., et al., Mycosis fungoides with recurrent Hodgkin's lymphoma and diffuse large B-cell lymphoma. *Acta Derm Venereol,* 2009. 89(4): p. 421-2.

[36] Goodlad, J., Calonje E, Brenn T, Lazar A, McKee PH, Cutaneous Limphoproliferative diseases and related disorders, in *McKee's Pathology of the Skin*. 4. ed. 2012, Saunders: Philadelphia. p. 1329-30.

[37] Teixeira, M., et al., Granulomatous slack skin. *Eur J Dermatol*, 2007. 17(5): p. 435-8.

[38] Ryan, E. A., et al., Can mycosis fungoides begin in the epidermis? A hypothesis. *Br J Dermatol*, 1973. 88(5): p. 419-29.

[39] Smith, N. P. and P. D. Samman, Mycosis fungoides presenting with areas of cutaneous hypopigmentation. *Clin Exp Dermatol*, 1978. 3(2): p. 213-6.

[40] Breathnach, S. M., P. H. McKee, and N. P. Smith, Hypopigmented mycosis fungoides: report of five cases with ultrastructural observations. *Br J Dermatol*, 1982. 106(6): p. 643-9.

[41] Zackheim, H. S., et al., Mycosis fungoides presenting as areas of hypopigmentation: a report of three cases. *J Am Acad Dermatol*, 1982. 6(3): p. 340-5.

[42] Amorim, G. M., et al., Hypopigmented mycosis fungoides: a 20-case retrospective series. *Int J Dermatol*, 2018. 57(3): p. 306-312.

[43] Alsaleh, Q. A., et al., Clinicoepidemiological features of mycosis fungoides in Kuwait, 1991-2006. *Int J Dermatol*, 2010. 49(12): p. 1393-8.

[44] Rodney, I. J., et al., Hypopigmented mycosis fungoides: a retrospective clinicohistopathologic study. *J Eur Acad Dermatol Venereol*, 2017. 31(5): p. 808-814.

[45] Stone, M. L., et al., Hypopigmented mycosis fungoides: a report of 7 cases and review of the literature. *Cutis*, 2001. 67(2): p. 133-8.

[46] Pavlovsky, L., et al., Hyperpigmented mycosis fungoides: an unusual variant of cutaneous T-cell lymphoma with a frequent CD8+ phenotype. *J Am Acad Dermatol*, 2012. 67(1): p. 69-75.

[47] David, M., et al., Diffuse, progressive hyperpigmentation: an unusual skin manifestation of mycosis fungoides. *J Am Acad Dermatol*, 1987. 16(1 Pt 2): p. 257-60.

[48] Lu, Y. Y., et al., Hyperpigmentation as a peculiar presentation of mycosis fungoides. *An Bras Dermatol*, 2017. 92(5 Suppl 1): p. 92-94.

[49] Jawed, S. I., et al., Primary cutaneous T-cell lymphoma (mycosis fungoides and Sézary syndrome): part I. Diagnosis: clinical and histopathologic features and new molecular and biologic markers. *J Am Acad Dermatol*, 2014. 70(2): p. 205.e1-16; quiz 221-2.

[50] Vonderheid, E. C., et al., Update on erythrodermic cutaneous T-cell lymphoma: report of the International Society for Cutaneous Lymphomas. *J Am Acad Dermatol,* 2002. 46(1): p. 95-106.

[51] Campbell, J. J., et al., Sézary syndrome and mycosis fungoides arise from distinct T-cell subsets: a biologic rationale for their distinct clinical behaviors. *Blood,* 2010. 116(5): p. 767-71.

[52] Kamijo, H. and M. Sugaya, Two distinct variants of mycosis fungoides (MF): Folliculotropic MF and erythrodermic MF. *J Dermatol*, 2019. 46(12): p. 1136-1140.

[53] Vonderheid, E. C., et al., A histo-immunopathologic and prognostic study of erythrodermic cutaneous T-cell lymphoma. *J Cutan Pathol,* 2019. 46(12): p. 913-924.

[54] Talpur, R., et al., Long-term outcomes of 1,263 patients with mycosis fungoides and Sézary syndrome from 1982 to 2009. *Clin Cancer Res,* 2012. 18(18): p. 5051-60.

[55] Abbott, R. A., et al., Poikilodermatous mycosis fungoides: a study of its clinicopathological, immunophenotypic, and prognostic features. *J Am Acad Dermatol*, 2011. 65(2): p. 313-319.

[56] Xu, P. and C. Tan, Dermoscopy of poikilodermatous mycosis fungoides (MF). *J Am Acad Dermatol*, 2016. 74(3): p. e45-7.

[57] Shiomi, T., et al., Poikilodermatous mycosis fungoides with a CD8+ CD56+ immunophenotype: a case report and literature review. *J Cutan Pathol,* 2013. 40(3): p. 317-20.

[58] Magro, C. M., et al., Cutaneous CD4+ CD56+ hematologic malignancies. *J Am Acad Dermatol,* 2010. 63(2): p. 292-308.

[59] Wain, E. M., et al., Outcome in 34 patients with juvenile-onset mycosis fungoides: a clinical, immunophenotypic, and molecular study. *Cancer,* 2003. 98(10): p. 2282-90.

In: Mycosis Fungoides and Sézary Syndrome ISBN: 978-1-68507-093-9
Editors: X. Zhang and L. Sokol

Chapter 7

MYCOSIS FUNGOIDES IN PEDIATRIC AND ADOLESCENT YOUNG ADULT PATIENTS

Eva Niklinska, MD
and Lucia Seminario-Vidal,* MD, PhD
Vanderbilt University Medical Center, Nashville, TN, USA
Department of Dermatology and Cutaneous Surgery,
University of South Florida Morsani College of Medicine,
Tampa, FL, USA
Department of Cutaneous Oncology,
H. Lee Moffitt Cancer Center and Research Institute, Tampa, FL, USA

INTRODUCTION

Amongst the myriad of conditions treated by pediatric dermatologists, a common patient presentation is that of hypopigmented patches. Ngo et al. reported a case of an eight-year-old Hispanic male who presented to clinic with hypopigmented patches on the lower legs, thighs, and buttocks. These patches had developed by six months of age, and they evolved over the past seven years. He was previously diagnosed with vitiligo; however,

* Corresponding Author's Email: luciasem@usf.edu.

biopsy revealed mycosis fungoides (MF) [1]. This case conveys a sentiment Ferreira et al. shared in their review, "Hypopigmented patches in childhood: do not forget mycosis fungoides" [2]. In order to keep the diagnosis of MF in the differential diagnosis of pediatricians, oncologists and dermatologists, we will highlight current MF literature for pediatric and adolescent young adult (AYA) patients regarding diagnosis, prognosis and treatment.

EPIDEMIOLOGY

MF is the most common cutaneous lymphoma in adults and children, constituting 65% of reported pediatric cutaneous lymphoma cases [3]. MF is more common in adults with an incidence of 0.64 per 100,000 persons per year [3]. In the United States, pediatric MF is rare with an incidence of 0.05 per 100 000 persons per year before 20 years of age and 0.12 per 100 000 persons per year for 20 - 29 years of age [4]. The prevalence of pediatric MF compared to adult-reported cases varies geographically with pediatric MF composing 4-5% of total MF cases in the United States, 16.6% of total MF cases in Kuwait, and 11% of total MF cases in Singapore [3, 5-7]. Importantly, MF targets populations of color. In adults greater than 30 years of age, MF has the highest incidence in Black patients; however, prevalence remains increased in Caucasian populations. In those under 30 years of age, including children and adolescents, MF has the highest prevalence in those of Asian, Pacific Islander or African American descent [4, 8].

Pediatric MF is extremely rare and its prevalence has not yet been calculated. Conversely, pediatric skin conditions that mimic MF are common. For example, vitiligo has a prevalence of 0.1- 1.8% [9], atopic dermatitis of 10-20% [10], and superficial fungal infections of 10-50% [11-13].

While much is known about MF in adults, pediatric MF literature remains sparse due to the low prevalence of the disease. In fact, it is based on a small number of studied cohorts with less than 500 reported and biopsy-confirmed pediatric MF patients to date, per our knowledge. Many of these cohorts included AYAs, such as those less than 21 years of age. The largest report of 71 pediatric patients comes out of Israel through the work of Dr. Emmilia Hodak [14]. Studied and reported cohorts >10 patients include*:

Table 7-1. Pediatric/AYA study cohorts > 10 patients

Study/Cohort Size	Country	Details
14 children [15]	Argentina	• *Age cutoff:* Not specified, all patients < 16 years of age. • *Race/Ethnicity:* Not specified, patient population from Argentina/Latin America.
20 children [16]	Turkey	• *Age cutoff:* ≤ 18 yo • *Race/Ethnicity:* Not specified, patient population from Turkey.
23 children [17]	Columbia	• *Age cutoff:* ≤ 18 yo • *Race/Ethnicity:* Not specified, patient population from Colombia.
23 children [18]	Korea	• *Age cutoff:* <20 yo • *Race/Ethnicity:* Not specified, patient population from South Korea.
24 children [19]	United States	• *Age cutoff:* ≤ 21 yo • This retrospective review included 24 patients who had symptom onset in childhood. Only 13 had biopsy-confirmed MF at ≤ 21 years of age. • *Race/Ethnicity:* Not specified, patient population from USA.
28 children [20]	Canada	• *Age cutoff:* ≤ 18 yo • *Race/Ethnicity:* Not specified, patient population from Canada. Patients classified by Fitzpatrick skin type.
30 children [21]	Iran	• *Age cutoff: Age cutoff:* ≤ 18 yo • *Race/Ethnicity:* Iranian (29), Afghan (1)
34 children [22]	United Kingdom	• *Age cutoff:* ≤ 16 yo • *Race/Ethnicity:* Not specified, patient population from UK.
34 children [23]	United States	• *Age cutoff:* ≤ 20 yo • *Race/Ethnicity:* Caucasian (10), African American (9), Hispanic (11), Indian (2), Middle Eastern (2)
36 children [6]	Kuwait	• *Age cutoff:* ≤ 18 yo • *Race/Ethnicity:* Arab (36)
46 children [24]	Singapore	• *Age cutoff:* ≤ 16 yo • *Race/Ethnicity:* Chinese (33), Malay (7), Indian (2), Other (4)
69 children [25]	United States	• *Age cutoff:* ≤ 21 yo • *Race/Ethnicity:* Caucasian (7), African American (39), Hispanic (17), Asian (6)
71 children [14]	Israel	• *Age cutoff:* ≤ 18 yo • *Race/Ethnicity:* Not specified, patient population from Israel.

* Cohorts from the same institution augmented over time through additional data are only included in their most recent form. **Race/ethnicity designations were directly copied from original article groupings/classifications.

Pediatric MF has a mean age at diagnosis of 10 years of age [24], with time to diagnosis of 2-5 years [26]. In concordance with adult presentations, lesions are most often found in sun-protected areas. The main types of pediatric MF are hypopigmented, folliculotropic, poikilodermatous, hyperpigmented, and classic (Fig. 7-1). Additional rare variants include granulomatous slack skin, granulomatous MF and pagetoid reticulosis.

CLINICAL SUBTYPES

MF Subtype	Diagnostic Pearls	Differential Diagnoses
Hypopigmented MF	*#1 most common peds presentation* • Hypopigmented patches / plaques ± scale • May exist in conjunction with classic erythematous lesions of MF • More common kin children with darker skin types (Fitzpatrick IV-VI)	• Pityriasis lichenoides • Atopic dermatitis • Vitiligo • Fungal infections • Pityriasis alba • Post-inflammatory hypopigmentation • Annular lichenoid dermatitis of youth (ALDY)
Folliculotropic MF	#2 most common peds presentation • Variable presentation • Localized alopecia within a lesion → erythematous plaque ± scale, follicular papules on erythematous base or hyperpigmentation overlaying skin changes (ie keratosis pilaris)	• Pityriasis rubra pilaris • Keratosis pilaris • Follicular mucinosis
Poikilodermatous MF	• Cutaneous atrophy, mottled skin and telangeictasias	• Acquired poikiloderma (ie manifestation of collagen vascular disease or radiation dermatitis)
Hyperpigmented MF	• Hyperpigmented patches • Frequently seen in combination with other MF variants	• Postinflammatory hyperpigmentation • Fixed drug eruption • Pigmented contact dermatitis • Ashy dermatosis • Lichen sclerosis • Idiopathic eruptive macular hyperpigmentation
Classic MF	• Erythematous, scaly patches / plaques	• Psoriasis • Atopic Dermatitis • Fixed drug eruptions • Fungal infections
Granulomatous Slack Skin (GSS)	• Lax, loose skin in major skin folds (axillae, groin)	• Cutis laxa • Intertrigo • Inverse psoriasis • Anetoderma
Granulomatous MF	• Nonscaly, thick plaques • May mimic benign granulomatous diseases (ie granuloma annulare, sarcoidosis or granulomatous rosacea)	• Benign granulomatous disease • Granuloma annulare • Sarcoid • Infectious granulomas
Pagetoid reticulosis	• Solitary, persistent, scaly plaque commonly on the limb	• Broad: papulosquamous, eczematoid, infectious, neoplastic diseases

Figure 7-1. Pediatric MF Subtypes, diagnostic pearls and potential differential diagnoses.

Hypopigmented MF

Hypopigmented MF is the most common pediatric presentation, accounting for more than 50% of pediatric MF cases [3, 14, 27]. The presentation can be isolated, multiple or confluent non-atrophic hypopigmented patches and plaques with or without fine overlaying scale or surrounding/superimposed erythema that may mask diagnosis (Fig. 7-2). It primarily affects Black and Asian children, with an average age of diagnosis of 17 years old [3]. Greater diagnosis in children with darker skin types (Fitzpatrick IV-VI) prompts the question of whether this variant is truly more prevalent in skin of color or underdiagnosed in children with fair skin [28]. Additionally, it is possible to have hypopigmented lesions in conjunction with the classic erythematous lesions of MF. This is an important consideration as children with both hypopigmented and classic MF lesions may experience more progressive disease to plaques/tumors than their counterparts with only hypopigmented lesions [25, 28, 29].

While classic MF shows a predominance of CD4+ T-cells, hypopigmented MF is characterized by a predominance of neoplastic and reactive CD8+ T-cells. Differential staining between neoplastic cells and tumor infiltrating lymphocytes (TILs) for granulysin has been reported. Neoplastic CD8+ CD7– cells often stained negatively for granulysin, while CD8+ CD7+ TILs were positive for granulysin [30]. It has been hypothesized that damage and alteration in melanocyte functions responsible for the hypopigmented lesions may be due to reactive TILs. This theory modulates hypopigmentation as a surrogate marker for an antitumor immune response, perhaps more prevalent in children due to their robust immune responses prior to immunosenescence [25]. On the other hand, it has been suggested that the cytotoxic effect of CD8+ T-cells is related to the pathogenesis of hypopigmented MF. CD8+T-cells influence melanocyte differentiation and melanogenesis through diminished expression of CD 117 (stem cell factor receptor/KIT protein) and melanocyte-specific microphthalmia-associated transcription factor. These interactions result in melanocytes loss which clinically presents as hypopigmentation [31].

As the pathogenesis of vitiligo is also related to destruction of melanocyte by the CD8+ T lymphocytes, it is important to differentiate these two conditions. Clinically, the presence of surface changes, such as scale or poikiloderma, presence of concomitant plaques or hyperpigmented lesions, favors hypopigmented MF. Histologically, epidermotropism, loss of CD7 expression, partial loss of pigment, preservation of some melanocytes, presence of lymphocytes within the papillary dermis, and increased density of the dermal infiltrate favors the diagnosis of hypopigmented MF over vitiligo [32].

Due to its variable presentation, a differential diagnosis for hypopigmented MF includes pityriasis lichenoides, atopic dermatitis, vitiligo, fungal infections, pityriasis alba, post-inflammatory hypopigmentation, and annular lichenoid dermatitis of youth (ALDY).

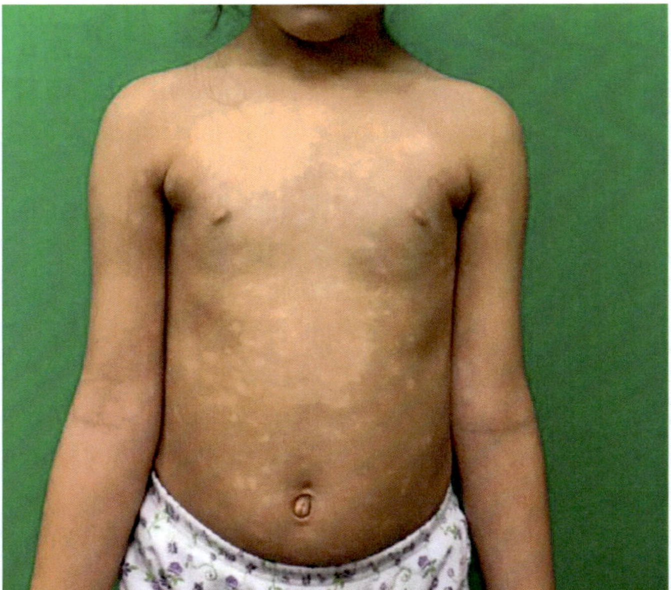

Figure 7-2. Hypopigmented MF. Multiple isolated and confluent, well-defined, hypopigmented patches on the trunk and extremities of a child.

Differential Diagnoses

Pityriasis lichenoides (PL) is an inflammatory dermatosis classified in two main variants, pityriasis lichenoides et varioliformis acuta (PLEVA), and the chronic variant, PLC [33]. Both PLEVA and PLC are difficult to diagnose and categorize. PLEVA is characterized by the sudden onset of erythematous macules that progress into papules with a fine scale [34]. A central vesiculopustular point with a hemorrhagic crust develops in most lesions and, as they heal, a varioliform scar forms [35]. PLC may present after PLEVA subsides or exist synchronously. PLC lesions can be distinguished from PLEVA by their slower development of small, dim, hypopigmented to erythematous or brownish macules or papules (Fig. 7-3) [34]. Although rare, systemic symptoms such as pruritus and fever may occur [36]. Histologically, hyperkeratosis and parakeratosis are seen in PL. In PLEVA, necrotic keratinocytes can be seen vacuolized in the basal layer, and there may be focal epidermal necrosis [36]. The dermis presents with edema and a lympho-histiocytic perivascular inflammatory infiltrate [36]. These infiltrates extend deep into the reticular dermis and are commonly wedge-shaped. Lymphocytes are usually CD8+ [34]. The blood vessels may also become affected by the inflammatory cells, resulting in vasculitis. Histology of PLC shows superficial CD4+ T cell-dominant lymphocytic infiltrates in a banded, perivascular distribution [34]. Keratinocytic necrosis, hemorrhage, neutrophilic infiltrate, spongiosis, and vesicle formation are rarely seen. In a study of 46 pediatric MF patients from Singapore, 46% were initially diagnosed and treated for PLC prior to biopsy-confirmed MF [24].

In a cohort of 34 pediatric patients with mycosis fungoides from the United States, greater than one third were initially diagnosed with atopic dermatitis (AD) [23]. Atopic dermatitis (Fig. 7-4) differs from hypopigmented MF in that it often presents in younger patients, with many children presenting within the first 6 months of life. Approximately 60% of cases present by one year of age and at least 85% of children with AD present by five years of age [37, 38]. AD is a clinical diagnosis based on chronicity, associated pruritus, and lesion distribution. Typical age-specific patterns include the face, neck and extensor surfaces in infants and children, compared to flexural surfaces in older children and adolescents (Fig. 7-4), with sparing of the axilla and groin [37]. Pediatric AD presents in three phases: (1) Infantile, characterized by erythematous papules/ patches, often in symmetrical distribution with edema, oozing and crusting independent of secondary infections; (2) Childhood (2 years of age – puberty), characterized by lichenified papules/plaques in extremities associated with severe pruritus; (3) Adult (age > puberty), characterized by dry, scaly, erythematous papules and plaques with associated lichenification [37]. In all stages, post-inflammatory hypopigmentation may occur. Additionally, children with AD commonly suffer from asthma and allergic rhinitis. As AD is a clinical diagnosis, it is not often biopsied. However, histopathology of AD would reveal nonspecific spongiotic dermatitis. In the acute phase, superficial perivascular lymphocytic infiltrate may be noted with occasional eosinophils. In subacute and chronic phases, additional parakeratosis, acanthosis and papillomatosis may be present [39].

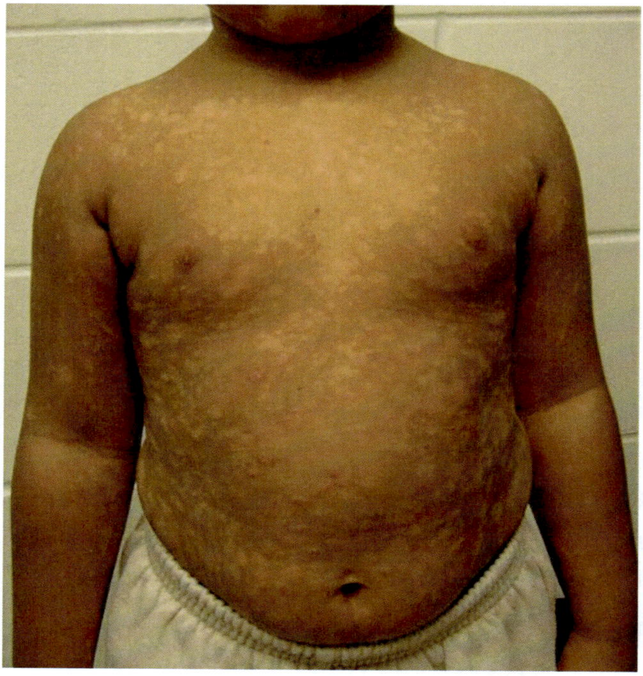

Figure 7-3. PLC. Erythematous scaly papules and hypopigmented scaly macules on trunk and extremities of a child.

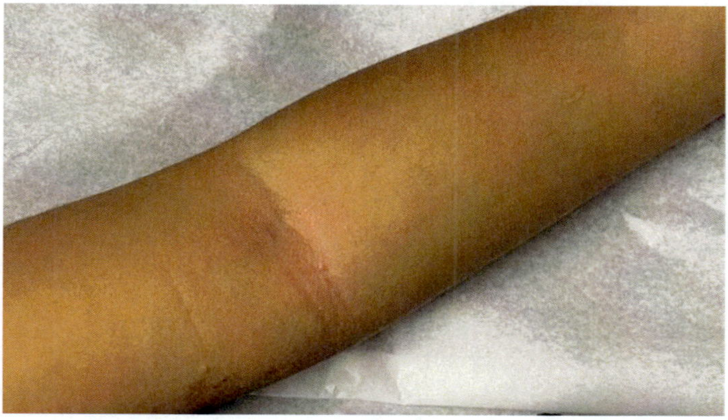

Figure 7-4. Atopic Dermatitis. Erythematous patch with excoriations and mild lichenification on the antecubital fossa.

Vitiligo, another mimicker of MF, is a disease of combined genetic predisposition and environmental triggers resulting in melanocyte destruction. Roughly one half of all cases begin in childhood with a slight female predominance in some studies [40, 41]. The average age of onset is 4-8 years old [41, 42]. Lesion manifestation may be segmental along embryonal development lines (lines of Blaschko), or nonsegmental (generalized) along skin folds, pressure points on hips/extremities, and perioral areas. (Fig. 7-5) Studies have found generalized vitiligo to be the most common presentation in children, followed by segmental and focal vitiligo [41-44]. Children are more likely to have segmental vitiligo than adults, and the age of onset is often earlier than other subtypes [42, 45]. Childhood vitiligo is also associated with positive family history, poliosis, and halo nevi [45]. Physical exam will reveal well-defined depigmented or hypopigmented patches with at least half of children having oral involvement [40]. To aid in diagnosis, Wood's lamp should be utilized to illuminate depigmented areas and dermoscopy can aid in assessing hair pigmentation reservoirs. Although not conventionally performed, histology would demonstrate absent pigment cells with or without inflammatory lymphocytes. S100 or MelanA stains can be utilized to compare pigment loss to control biopsy from adjacent normal skin [46]. As abovementioned, the clinical and histological presentations are helpful in differentiating vitiligo from hypopigmented MF.

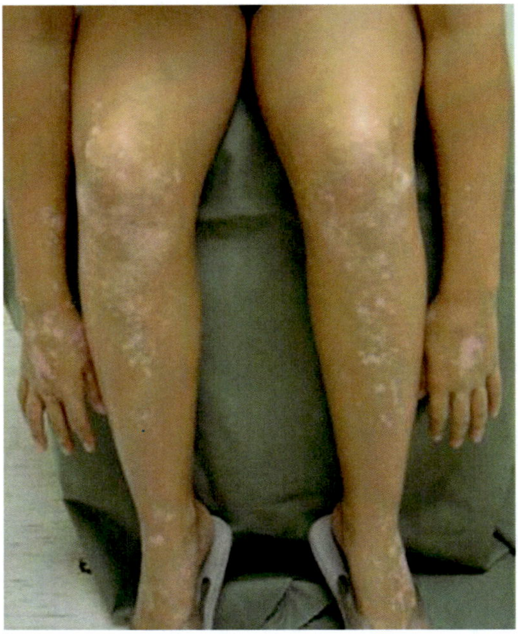

Figure 7-5. Vitiligo. Generalized solitary and confluent depigmented patches on the extensor surfaces of extremities in a child.

Tinea versicolor (TV), also known as pityriasis versicolor, is a superficial mycosis caused by the yeast and fungi of the genus Malassezia, which comes in three dominant species: *M furfur, M globosa, and M sympodialis.* The clinical presentation of tinea versicolor is defined by hypochromic or hyperchromic solitary and coalescing macules and patches with fine overlaying scale. (Fig. 7-6) The macules/patches are generally found on the trunk and upper extremities, with greater facial involvement in children [47]. Predisposing factors for the development of TV are humidity, heat (summer months), hyperhidrosis, oral contraceptives, application of oils/serums and treatment with topical corticosteroids [48]. Although TV is usually asymptomatic, it can be associated with pruritus. Diagnosis is clinical, and the presence of fine scale overlaying macules/patches is augmented upon stretching the skin (Zileri's sign) or with fine scraping [48]. Wood's lamp testing reveals a yellow, golden fluorescence and fine scaling can also be seen via dermoscopy [49]. KOH testing with the classic "spaghetti and meatballs" of thick pseudohyphae and blastospore clusters

[50]. Biopsy is rarely performed; however, when undertaken it could reveal follicular abnormalities (such as atrophy and degeneration), as well as mild hyperkeratosis and acanthosis [48].

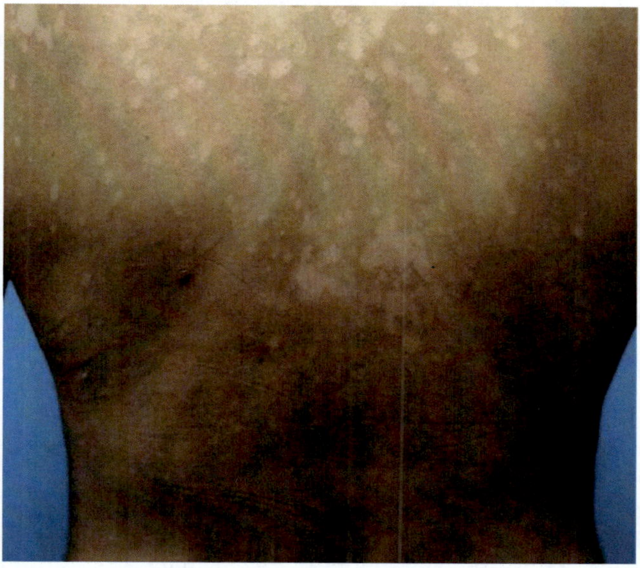

Figure 7-6. Tinea versicolor. Isolated and coalescing hypopigmented macules and patches on the upper back of an adolescent. Closer inspection reveals mild overlying scale.

In close relationship to tinea (pityriasis) versicolor is pityriasis alba (PA), another potential mimicker of MF. The classic clinical presentation of this multistage disease is ill-defined erythematous macules/patches that subside and result in areas of hypopigmentation with scaling edges. The etiology of PA is multifactorial and the disease presents as long-term with frequent, spontaneous remissions. In early lesions, histopathology is notable for irregular melanin pigmentation of the basal epidermal later, sebaceous gland atrophy, and keratotic hair follicle blockage [51].

Post-inflammatory hypopigmentation (PIH) is another critical diagnosis to consider in the differential for MF. PIH occurs due to exogenous or endogenous trauma to the skin, including the resolution of other dermatologic inflammatory conditions. While it occurs in all skin types, it may be more noticeable in darker skin tones. Clinical diagnosis requires investigation into other underlying disease processes/trauma, and histology is nonspecific with decreased epidermal melanin, melanophages in the upper dermis, and variable lymphohistiocytic infiltration [52].

Annular lichenoid dermatitis of youth (ALDY) is a subtype of lichenoid dermatoses, described by Annessi et al. in 2003. The mean age of diagnosis is 11 years old, with the eruption of 1+ well-defined erythematous macules [53]. Over time, the macules extend to form large, annular plaques with raised erythematous borders and central areas of hypopigmentation. Eruptions have a predilection for the groin or flank. The patches of ALDY can be differentiated from MF due to their pigmented borders and lack of wrinkly surface [53]. In addition to clinical recognition, biopsy can guide diagnosis. In early disease stages, histology reveals band-like largely lymphocytic infiltrates in the papillary dermis with vacuolar alteration in the dermal-epidermal junction. In later stages, the lymphocytes move to the rete ridge tips causing major keratinocyte necrosis/apoptosis. This will ultimately lead to an epidermis devoid of rete ridges due to keratinocyte damage [53, 54]. The epidermotropic lymphocytes express CD8; however, the perivascular infiltrates are CD4 predominant [54]. While vacuolar changes have been noted in MF biopsies (especially those with poikilodermatous change), the most important histologic factor distinguishing ALDY from MF is the presence of necrotic/apoptotic keratinocyte clusters strictly at the tips of the rete ridges [53]. MF has many overlapping clinical and histological characteristics with ALDY and is increasingly difficult to differentiate.

Folliculotropic MF

The second most common form of pediatric MF is folliculotropic (FMF), accounting for up to 39-42% of cases [14, 27]. It is characterized by localized alopecia within a lesion. It can present as an erythematous plaque with or without scale [55, 56], follicular papules on an erythematous base [3], or hyperpigmentation overlaying additional skin changes such as keratosis pilaris [57]. Additional manifestations may include grouped follicular/acneiform papules, comedones, pustules, milia or indurated plaques and tumors [58]. In a cohort study by Hodak et al. where FMF accounted for 36% of cases, the majority of patients had a combination of hypopigmented and typical FMF lesions [27].

Differential diagnosis includes pityriasis rubra pilaris, keratosis pilaris, and follicular mucinosis (argued by some scholars to be a precursor or overlap of follicular MF) [3, 55].

Differential Diagnoses

Pityriasis rubra pilaris (PRP) is a rare idiopathic papulosquamous inflammatory disorder classified into 6 types, with types III-V describing childhood manifestations. Type III, also known as Classic Juvenile PRP, presents around 5-10 years of age with an acute onset of red-orange keratotic follicular papules which coalesce into plaques with characteristic islands of sparing [59]. These plaques usually affect the upper body, especially the face/neck. Additional clinical manifestations may include erythroderma, palmoplantar keratoderma, and nail changes (rough, thickened, yellow) [59]. Children with type III PRP have a good prognosis, with most lesions spontaneously resolving within one year [60]. Type IV (Circumscribed Juvenile) manifests as sharply demarcated areas of follicular hyperkeratosis and erythema over the elbows and knees in prepubertal children. Transient scaly macules may be seen over other bony prominences, and its prognosis is less favorable [59]. Type V (Atypical Juvenile), which usually includes most familial cases of PRP, has an early onset and long disease course with follicular hyperkeratosis presentation and scleratodermous changes of the hands/feet [59]. Diagnosis is guided by clinical presentation and histopathology. Histology is notable for psoriasiform dermatitis with irregular hyperkeratosis and a characteristic "checkerboard pattern" consisting of alternating horizontal and vertical orthokeratosis and parakeratosis [61]. Focal or confluent hypergranulosis may be seen with sparse superficial perivascular infiltrate in the dermis, and thick suprapapillary plates [59]. Additionally, acantholysis and focal acantholytic dyskeratosis have been described, which may aid differentiation from psoriasis [61].

Keratosis pilaris (KP) is a common, inherited hyperkeratotic disorder characterized by grouped, small, folliculocentric keratotic papules with surrounding erythema [62]. Due to their stippled appearance, the papules may resemble gooseflesh. The classic distribution of this benign condition is over the extensor surfaces of the upper arms, upper thighs and buttocks [63]. KP presents within the first decade of life for half of patients, and is usually asymptomatic, although it may be associated with pruritus. KP also has seasonal variation with patients reporting wintertime exacerbation [63]. While diagnosis is largely clinical, histology would reveal excess keratin as horny plugs resulting in a dilated follicular infundibulum. Mild, superficial lymphohistiocytic infiltrate may be noted in the upper dermis and perifollicular areas [62].

Follicular mucinosis (FM) is a rare cutaneous disease with unknown etiology which has often been described as closely related to FMF due to similar presentation. FM is characterized by an acute/subacute eruption of hypopigmented, eczematous plaques and/or flesh-colored, follicular papules on the head/neck [55]. The concurrence of FM and FMF varies widely among studies (9.4-60%) [55], and controversy exists whether FM is a clonal inflammatory process or a neoplastic process serving as an MF precursor. Differentiating between FM and FMF can be challenging histologically [64]. FM histology includes mucin deposition within the external root sheath, infundibulum and sebaceous glands, marked follicular dilation, and presence of mixed perifollicular infiltrate with lymphocytes, histiocytes and eosinophils [65]. If concurrent MF is present, cytologically atypical or cerebriform lymphocytes and a band-like lymphocytic infiltrate will be noted. In one study of 11 pediatric patients, FM was not found to be equivalent to MF. Only 3 patients had histopathologic findings consistent with MF and all were diagnosed on initial biopsy [55]. Another study of 31 children found that 90% of subject biopsies demonstrated some degree of folliculotropism, 50% of biopsies demonstrated epidermotropism and 35% of cases had a mild degree of nuclear atypia. Although 12 of these cases met the score limit of 4 on International Society of Cutaneous Lymphomas algorithm diagnostic criteria for early MF diagnosis [66], only 2 had histopathologic findings typical of MF [65]. Based on this data, Zvulonov et al. recommended that the ISCL diagnostic algorithm should exclude children with FM [65]. Due to remaining uncertainty, close follow-up may be warranted for pediatric FM patients [3].

Other MF Variants

Hyperpigmented MF composes up to 29% of pediatric MF cases (based on a study of 34 patients) [23]. It is characterized by hyperpigmented patches/plaques with varying degrees of atrophy, scaling, and irregular border definition [67]. It is frequently seen in combination with other MF variants, and in adults, is overrepresented in patients with skin of color [68]. However, due to the presence of hyperpigmentation in many inflammatory cutaneous processes, it is difficult to determine the true prevalence of hyperpigmented MF. A potential differential diagnosis for hyperpigmented MF includes postinflammatory hyperpigmentation, fixed drug eruption, pigmented contact dermatitis, ashy dermatosis, morphea, and idiopathic eruptive macular hyperpigmentation [67].

Poikilodermatous MF composes up to 26% of juvenile MF cases (based on a study of 34 patients) and presents with cutaneous atrophy, mottled skin and telangeictasias [3, 23]. In adults, this variant is commonly found on the breast, hips, and buttocks. A differential diagnosis includes acquired poikiloderma due to collagen vascular disease or radiation dermatitis [67].

Classic MF, notable for erythematous patches/plaques with overlying scale, is cited in approximately 40% of cases, most often in older children [14, 23, 69]. A differential diagnosis includes psoriasis, atopic dermatitis, fixed drug eruptions, and fungal infections.

Granulomatous slack skin (GSS*)* is a rare variant characterized by progressive development of lax, loose skin in major skin folds, preferentially the axillae and groin. These lesions begin as hardened, erythematous plaques that pedunculate with time. <5 pediatric cases have been described in the literature [70-72]. While multiple treatment modalities have been utilized, treatment outcomes are often disappointing. Differential diagnosis for GSS includes cutis laxa, intertrigo, inverse psoriasis and anetoderma.

Granulomatous MF is a rare subtype with few (<10) reported pediatric cases [73-77]. Clinical features may include nonscaly, thick plaques without the pendulous skin characteristic of granulomatous slack skin disease. Granulomatous MF may mimic benign granulomatous diseases such as granuloma annulare, sarcoidosis or granulomatous rosacea [67]. While granulomatous MF confers worse prognostic outcomes in adults, there is limited data for pediatric patients.

Pagetoid reticulosis (PR) is a rare variant of MF in both adults and children. Also known as Woringer-Kolopp disease, this variant was first reported in 1939 by the two researchers for which it is named. Since the original case, there are less than 10 reported cases, as far as we are aware, in the literature [78-82]. It is characterized by a solitary, persistent, scaly plaque commonly on the limb. Pagetoid reticulosis, due to its solitary lesion appearance, has often been described hand in hand with unilesional MF. *Unilesional MF* is emerging as a newly recognized MF entity, characterized by a single erythematous patch with overlaying scale [83]. A retrospective review of pediatric MF cases from one referral center in Turkey found that 20% of children presented with unilesional MF [16]. While unilesional MF is histopatologically identical to classic MF, [84] PR is differentiated from unilesional MF by (1) marked hyperkeratosis, (2) pagetoid epidermotropism, and (3) dermal infiltrate lacking eosinophils [82].

Diagnosis

Diagnosis of pediatric MF follows adult-established guidelines focused on clinical recognition with biopsy-supported pathology. Please refer to Chapters 3-5 for adult diagnostic pathways and pathologic features. Pediatric/AYA patient evaluation begins with a complete physical exam as well as documentation of % BSA and skin lesion morphology (often with the help of clinical photos). Regional lymph nodes and organs should be palpated to assess for lymphadenopathy or organomegaly [28] (Table 7-7).

As previously described, there is a wide range of differential diagnoses associated with each MF subtype. If the patient history and clinical presentation correlate most strongly with a benign skin condition, it is acceptable to try first-line therapies for the presumably benign skin condition. However, it is crucial to remain alert and assess the patient regularly for worsening symptoms or failure to respond to therapy, which may prompt a further diagnostic pathway. If the patient's history and presentation due not strongly align with a benign condition, a biopsy is warranted. Children have greater skin sensitivity and potential for scarring; thus, biopsy approach must be taken with care.

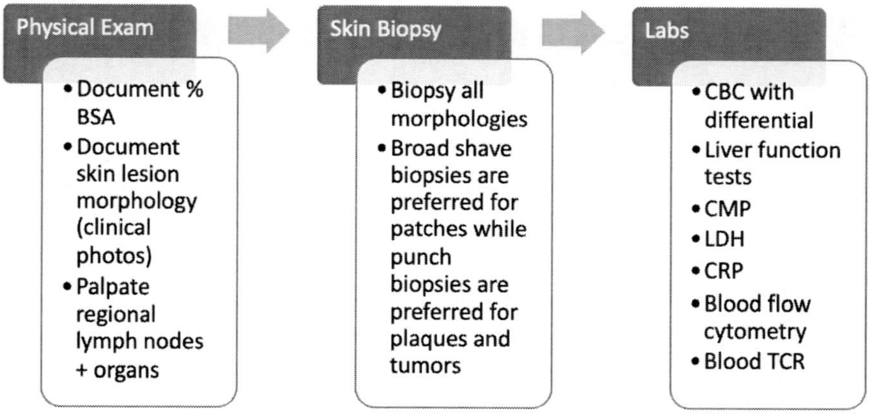

Figure 7-7. Initial pediatric MF workup.

For evaluation of suspicious lesions in pediatric and AYA patients, we generally recommend to biopsy all morphologies. Broad shave biopsies are helpful in evaluating more epidermis and they are preferred for patches. Punch biopsies are recommended for evaluation of folliculotropism and they are preferred for plaques, and tumors. Punch biopsies include deep tissue layers and cause less scarring. Established lesions with the most primary change should be chosen over new lesions which may be nonspecific. Importantly, the lines of least skin tension (Langer lines) should be identified surrounding the intended biopsy site. The skin should be stretched 90 degrees perpendicular to the Langer lines in order to promote an elliptical lesion with easier, linear closure. Biopsy sties can be closed with 1-2 interrupted nylon sutures. 5-0 nylon is utilized for most nonfacial areas, with

6-0 nylon utilized for the face. Recall that topical steroids must be discontinued 2-3 weeks prior to biopsy as they may blunt MF histologic features. Furthermore, a careful drug history is crucial prior to biopsy due to potential mimicry from early drug eruptions [85].

To supplement the skin biopsy, initial bloodwork may be warranted, including: CBC with differential, liver function tests, CMP, LDH and CRP. If SS is suspected or patients present with advanced stages or rare variants, blood work should also include TCR gene rearrangement studies and Sézary cell count/blood flow cytometry. In these patients, imaging studies should be also performed to evaluate for lymph node involvement [86].

Upon pathologic review of the biopsy tissue with concordant immunohistochemistry (IHC), neoplastic T-cells in MF present as the helper (CD3+, CD4+, CD8-) or cytotoxic (CD3+, CD4-, CD98+) variety. Key pathologic characteristics for recognition include (1) atypical, cerebriform T-cells, (2) lymphoid infiltrate in superficial papillary dermis, (3) epidermotropism and (4) Pautrier microabscesses [87]. Certain MF subtypes may have more specific histopathologic changes:

- Hypopigmented MF: epidermotropism of small-to-medium lymphocytes. IHC shows reduced CD7 staining [25]. Hypopigmented MF commonly shows a CD8+ phenotype, compared to classic MF's CD4+ phenotype.
- Folliculotropic MF: Neoplastic lymphocytic infiltration of the hair follicles ± epidermotropism [27]. In contrast to classic MF, interfollicular dermis is spared and Pautrier's microabcesses are infrequent [28].
- Poikilodermatous MF: atrophy of stratum basale and stratum spinosum, hydropic degeneration of the basal cell layer, melanophages in the papillary dermis, telangiectatic vessels [3].
- Granulomatous slack skin: CD68+ multinucleated giant cells and loss of elastic tissue [88].
- Granulomatous MF: granulomatous infiltrate of atypical lymphocytes (clonal Tcells), histiocytes, and multinucleated giant cells [73].

- Pagetoid reticulosis: marked Tcell epidermotropism with hyperkeratitis acanthosis. Variable immunophenotype with CD4+, CD8+ or CD4-/CD8- predominance [89].

In the presence of a strong clinical suspicion and equivocal biopsy result, flow cytometry may also be used to identify TCR gene rearrangement. It is important to recall that clonality garnered from flow cytometry does not equate to malignancy, as many benign conditions have reactive clonal populations [3, 90]. In pediatric MF diagnosis, the presence of clonality can vary. A recent study by Hodak et al. demonstrated monoclonal TCR in less than half (~43%) of children with FMF [27].

The immunophenotype in pediatric CTCL, such as MF, can be variable. While the majority of malignant T cells in adult CTCL are derived from CD4+ memory T cells, studies report an increased CD8+ phenotype in children [22]. In IHC analysis of 32 pediatric patients (≤ 16 years old), 63% had a CD4+ predominant phenotype, while 34% had a CD8+ predominant phenotype and 3% (1/32) had a CD8-/CD56+ phenotype [22]. This compares to less than 5% of adult cases with a cytotoxic immunophenotype. While CD8+ phenotypes are often connected to hypopigmented MF, unique cases have also demonstrated CD8+ CD56+ poikilodermatous MF in pediatric patients [91, 92]. Additionally, unlike in adults, the CD8+ phenotype does not appear to portend a poor prognosis [93].

Once the diagnosis is confirmed, clinical and TNMB staging guidelines follow those laid out for adults, as described in Chapter 11. Most children are diagnosed at Stage 1A/1B with patches and plaques but no tumor involvement [23]. For children with limited skin involvement (T1 N0 B0 or T2 N0 B0), chest x-ray and ultrasound of the abdomen and regional lymph nodes should be sufficient [93]. CT chest/abdomen/pelvis should be obtained in children with > Stage 1A and in some patients with limited T2 disease [93]. FDG-PET may be recommended to evaluate lymphadenopathy and potential organ involvement. For lymph nodes >1.5cm, or with firm or irregular features, excisional biopsy may be warranted with specimen pathologic assessment, TCR gene rearrangement, flow cytometry. Bone marrow biopsy is no longer considered essential for evaluation of all cases;

however, it should be considered for patients with extracutaneous involvement and SS [93]. Aggressive cases of pediatric MF have been described, and uniquely connected with underlying genetic germline mutations [94]. Therefore, following staging guidelines is critical, and may involve further testing.

Sézary Syndrome and Large Cell Transformation

Sézary Syndrome

Sézary Syndrome (SS) is the leukemic counterpart to MF. It is defined by diffuse erythroderma and a significant number of circulating malignant Sézary cells. SS is associated with pruritus, alopecia, and generalized lymphadenopathy. Histopathology from skin biopsy is often nondiagnostic, and peripheral blood flow cytometry, as well as bone marrow analysis, may be required for diagnosis and staging. Only isolated cases of pediatric Sézary syndrome have been reported [95-97]. Alberti-Violetti et al. described the case of a 17-year-old male diagnosed with SS [95]. His genomic analysis revealed chromosomal alterations consistent with previously described adult-onset SS, including losses on chromosome 10q and the presence of isochromosome 17q [98-100]. These changes coincide with suspected induction of deregulated proliferation (17q gain of function mutations of STAT3 and STAT5) and loss of proapoptotic genes (PTEN on 10q) contributing, together, to uncontrolled cell survival [98, 99]. Diagnostic and treatment guidelines follow adult recommendations.

Large Cell Transformation

In adults, approximately 20% of low-stage MF and SS undergo secondary transformation [101]. Large cell transformation (LCT) is characterized by $\geq$ 25% of clonally identical large cells in the dermal infiltrate. While rare, few pediatric cases of LCT-MF have been reported. One example includes the case of a pediatric patient with underlying BRCA-2 mutation who was diagnosed with large cell transformation of MF [94, 102-105]. The possibility of LCT should be kept in mind for pediatric patients who present with new onset tumors, do not respond to standard therapies or show disease progression. Like adult patients with CTCL, pediatric patients should be biopsied and re-staged if LCT is confirmed.

PROGNOSIS

Similar to adults, the number one prognostic factor for pediatric MF is extracutaneous involvement [3]. However, there is a scarcity of studies exploring long-term progression and outcomes in pediatric patients. In regard to prognosis, hypopigmented and poikilodermatous MF have been noted as contributing to favorable prognoses; age at diagnosis is equivocal; and folliculotropic MF has been suggested as unfavorable based on adult data [3, 22, 106]. However, newer studies have demonstrated that FMF can be divided into two clinical groups (indolent, advanced) with differing prognostic outcomes. The indolent group of follicle-based patches, flat plaques and acneiform lesions has a more favorable prognostic profile than the advanced group of thick follicle-based infiltrates and tumors which is less responsive to therapies [28, 107-111]. Unilesional MF has been associated with an excellent prognosis [83].

In a review of current literature and 366 pediatric MF cases, Wohlmuth-Wieser reported that only 5% of patients had advanced disease [28]. In this same analysis, 1% of cases lead to death. Therefore, due to a limited number of pediatric MF cases with extracutaneous involvement, it is difficult to draw any correlation or conclusions from TCR clonality and potential prognostic predictions [23]. In a population-based study of approximately 400 patients diagnosed with MF before 30 years of age, Ai et al. found that these patients had higher risks of secondary cancers (especially lymphoma and melanoma) [4]. Data supports the need for close pediatric MF patient follow-up throughout their lifetime.

Despite the rarity of MF in the pediatric and AYA population, there have been reported geographic clusters of adult MF patients through multiple studies in Sweden [112], the United States (Texas [113], Pennsylvania [114]), and Canada [115]. These groupings may suggest contributing and cumulative environmental exposures [116]. In fact, the Canadian study found CTCL clustering in heavy industrial areas, while areas with limited industrial presence were relatively spared [115]. In addition to considering heavy industry areas, data suggests that exposure to chemicals (such as pesticides), air pollution, and certain detergents may increase one's risk of developing MF, SS, and non-Hodgkin lymphomas [117, 118]. However, there is a lack of literature about environmental factors in connection with pediatric MF. With a potential cumulative nature, one could postulate that exposure to environmental toxins may not play as active of a role in pediatric MF development as MF developed later in adulthood.

In addition to geographic clusters, one must consider familial clusters and occurrences as combinations of environmental and genetic exposures. In additional to multiple cases involving first-degree relatives [119-123], Hodak et al. reported a cluster of 6 Jewish families (12 MF patients total) [124]. HLA analysis of the families revealed no specific haplotype, HLA class I antigen, or HLA-DR allele predominant. However, the DQB1*03 allele was found to be significantly increased compared to control. In this cohort, 2/12 patients were pediatric (<18 yo). In addition, a case report was published on two pediatric siblings (14 yo, 10 yo), diagnosed with MF [125]. Taken together with HLA data published on adults, this may suggest that there is a genetic predisposition or susceptibility for developing MF. However, further research is necessary to elucidate specific genes and pathways.

Potential genetic predispositions also beg the question of whether pediatric MF patients have an increased risk of certain comorbidities or familial cancer syndromes. A study of 74 patients diagnosed with MF prior to 30 years of age, Virmani et al. found that 8% had a family history of leukemia/lymphoma and 3% had other comorbid leukemias or lymphomas. In addition, 11% suffered from asthma and 5% from eczema [69]. In regard to familial cancer syndromes and pediatric MF comorbidities, future research is necessary to best understand the pathogenesis, interactions, and subsequent prognosis, of this disease.

Treatment

There are no established treatment protocols for pediatric patients with CTCL and therefore the therapeutic approach to childhood MF is similar to adults. Given that most pediatric MF patients are diagnosed in the 1A/1B stage, treatment focuses on skin-directed modalities. In their analysis of 248 pediatric MF cases from the literature, Wu et al. reviewed the most common treatment regimens for pediatric MF based on all English case series (>3 patients) between 2008-2018 [3]. The most prevalent treatment was phototherapy, including narrowband UVB (NBUVB) and psoralen and ultraviolet A (PUVA). About 77% of patients had at least partial response to phototherapy, with 36% of patients reporting complete symptom resolution. A lower response was noted in folliculotropic MF (FMF), perhaps due to follicular involvement. However, recent data suggest that FMF is more responsive to PUVA over NBUVB [14]. Wu et al. evaluated the need for additional phototherapy at 58% for NBUVB at 4 months and 50% for PUVA at 45.5 months [20]. Despite its well-documented treatment benefits, a special consideration must be given for the association of psoralen with cataracts, and preventative measures must be taken for children undergoing this treatment [126]. Of note, PUVA is associated with greater risk of nonmelanoma skin cancer development [93]. Overall, these results support previous research demonstrating higher rates of remission with PUVA, but safer therapeutic indices with NBUVB [127]. Taken together, the data may support NBUVB as a first-line treatment, with PUVA used for refractory cases [128]; however, the benefit of therapy must be weighed against the risks.

Additional treatments used either in isolation or conjunction with phototherapy included topical corticosteroids, topical retinoids, interferon and topical chemotherapies. Combination therapies yielded more optimal treatment responses. In the largest pediatric MF case series of 71 patients, Hodak et al. found a complete response rate of 75% after an average of 1.73 treatment modalities with no difference in response rates between folliculotropic and non-folliculotropic groups [14]. With an average follow-up period of 7.7 years, 83% of the cohort had at least one relapse [14]. In a review of 40 children, adolescents and young adults (mean age 29.2), Hooper et al. found that patients with advanced-stage MF received various first line therapies including topical nitrogen mustard, systemic steroids, systemic retinoids, radiation, PUVA or CHOP chemotherapy [129].

In regard to any treatment undertaken, therapeutic safety is even more crucial in pediatric patients than in adults due to children's susceptibility and future growth trajectories. Systemic chemotherapy should be avoided, is possible. Total skin electron beam therapy should be avoided, if possible. Systemic steroids should be limited due to negative impact on growth and potential osteoradionecrosis. There is a risk of premature bone growth stunting in young patients and risk of teratogenicity in AYAs with use of systemic retinoids. Additionally, there is a risk of bone marrow suppression with nitrogen mustard. Finally, although it is one of the most used and first line categories, topical steroids present a localized risk of skin atrophy, striae, perioral dermatitis, acne, and purpura.

It is important to note that while pediatric guidelines are limited, children are often treated "off-label" based on adult treatment algorithms and trials. For example, adults in stage 1A (limited patch/plaque) also utilize skin-directed therapies such as topical corticosteroids, topical mechlorethamine, topical bexarotene and NBUVB/PUVA. In stage IB, IIA adults receive therapies such as photopheresis, bexarotene capsules and vorinostat capsules are introduced [130, 131]. For adults with tumors (IIB), erythroderma (III) and blood/visceral involvement (IVA, B) systemic therapies may also include electron beam therapy, romidepsin, brentuximab, pralatrexate, mogalizumab (CCR4), single agent chemotherapy and hematopoetic stem cell transplant. Use of novel FDA-approved biological therapy, such as mentioned in adults, has not been validated in clinical trials with pediatric patients. These modalities require further exploration in pediatric patients through clinical trials and case reports. Currently, there are no clinical trials specific to pediatric mycosis fungoides/Sézary syndrome. However, trials for pediatric patients with recurrent/refractory solid tumors and leukemia are open to pediatric patients with recurrent mycosis fungoides or Sézary syndrome.

While much of treatment is targeted at the underlying MF, it is important to alleviate patient symptoms of pruritis and discomfort. For this concern, guidelines from atopic dermatitis treatment pathways can be followed. Both local and systemic medications are utilized for the treatment of pruritis. Local pruritis can be alleviated through use of emollients, wet wrap therapy and topical medications. Local medications include topical corticosteroids and topical calcineurin inhibitors (i.e., tacrolimus), topical phosphodiesterase 4 inhibitors (i.e., Crisaborole), topical analgesics and topical cooling agents (i.e., menthol). Oral medications used to alleviate pruritis include antihistamines, cyclosporine, methotrexate, corticosteroids, and biologic agents such as dupilumab. Each of these treatment modalities carries additional risks and needs to be weighed against benefit prior to start of therapy.

Conclusion

Pediatric MF remains a very rare condition with relatively good prognosis; however, its recognition, early treatment, and continuous monitoring for potential progression remain critical. We urge all physicians to maintain MF on their differential for pediatric and adolescent young adult patients with refractory or evolving presentations of common dermatoses.

References

[1] Ngo, J.T., M.J. Trotter, and R.M. Haber, Juvenile-onset hypopigmented mycosis fungoides mimicking vitiligo. *Journal of cutaneous medicine and surgery,* 2009. 13(4): p. 230-233.

[2] Ferreira, B., et al., Hypopigmented patches in childhood: do not forget mycosis fungoides. *Clinical and Experimental Dermatology,* 2019. 44(5): p. 588-589.

[3] Wu, J.H., B.A. Cohen, and R.J. Sweren, Mycosis fungoides in pediatric patients: Clinical features, diagnostic challenges, and advances in therapeutic management. *Pediatric dermatology,* 2020. 37(1): p. 18-28.

[4] Ai, W.Z., et al., Outcomes after diagnosis of mycosis fungoides and Sézary syndrome before 30 years of age: a population-based study. *JAMA dermatology,* 2014. 150(7): p. 709-715.

[5] Fink-Puches, R., et al., The spectrum of cutaneous lymphomas in patients less than 20 years of age. *Pediatric dermatology,* 2004. 21(5): p. 525-533.

[6] Nanda, A., et al., Mycosis fungoides in Arab children and adolescents: a report of 36 patients from Kuwait. *Pediatric Dermatology,* 2010. 27(6): p. 607-613.

[7] Tan, E., Y.K. Tay, and Y.C. Giam, Profile and outcome of childhood mycosis fungoides in Singapore. *Pediatric dermatology,* 2000. 17(5): p. 352-356.

[8] Criscione, V.D. and M.A. Weinstock, Incidence of cutaneous T-cell lymphoma in the United States, 1973-2002. *Archives of dermatology,* 2007. 143(7): p. 854-859.

[9] Mohr, N., et al., Epidemiology of Vitiligo–A Dual Population-Based Approach. *Clinical Epidemiology,* 2021. 13: p. 373.

[10] Nutten, S., Atopic dermatitis: global epidemiology and risk factors. *Annals of nutrition and metabolism,* 2015. 66(Suppl. 1): p. 8-16.

[11] Male, O., The significance of mycology in medicine. *Frontiers in Mycology.* Wallingford: CAB International, 1990: p. 131-156.

[12] Ameen, M., Epidemiology of superficial fungal infections. *Clinics in dermatology,* 2010. 28(2): p. 197-201.

[13] Seebacher, C., J.-P. Bouchara, and B. Mignon, Updates on the epidemiology of dermatophyte infections. *Mycopathologia,* 2008. 166(5-6): p. 335-352.

[14] Hodak, E., et al., Pediatric mycosis fungoides: Management and outcomes with special focus on the folliculotropic variant. *European Journal of Cancer,* 2018. 101: p. S33-S34.

[15] Cervini, A., et al., Mycosis fungoides: experience in a pediatric hospital. *Actas Dermo-Sifiliográficas* (English Edition), 2017. 108(6): p. 564-570.

[16] Yazganoglu, K., et al., Childhood mycosis fungoides: a report of 20 cases from Turkey. *Journal of the European Academy of Dermatology and Venereology,* 2013. 27(3): p. 295-300.

[17] Ocampo, O.V., et al., Mycosis Fungoides in Children and Adolescents: A Series of 23 Cases. *Actas Dermo-Sifiliográficas* (English Edition), 2020.

[18] KIM, S.T., et al., Clinicopathological features and T-cell receptor gene rearrangement findings of mycosis fungoides in patients younger than age 20 years. *The Journal of dermatology,* 2009. 36(7): p. 392-402.

[19] Zackheim, H.S., et al., Mycosis fungoides with onset before 20 years of age: review of 24 patients and report of a case diagnosed at age 22 months. *Journal of the American Academy of Dermatology,* 1997. 36(4): p. 557-562.

[20] Laws, P.M., N.H. Shear, and E. Pope, Childhood mycosis fungoides: experience of 28 patients and response to phototherapy. *Pediatric Dermatology,* 2014. 31(4): p. 459-464.

[21] Nasimi, M., et al., Childhood mycosis fungoides: A clinicopathologic study of 30 cases from Iran. *The Australasian journal of dermatology,* 2019.

[22] Wain, E.M., et al., Outcome in 34 patients with juvenile-onset mycosis fungoides: a clinical, immunophenotypic, and molecular study. *Cancer: Interdisciplinary International Journal of the American Cancer Society,* 2003. 98(10): p. 2282-2290.

[23] Boulos, S., et al., Clinical presentation, immunopathology, and treatment of juvenile-onset mycosis fungoides: a case series of 34 patients. *Journal of the American Academy of Dermatology,* 2014. 71(6): p. 1117-1126.

[24] Heng, Y.K., et al., Pediatric mycosis fungoides in Singapore: a series of 46 children. *Pediatric dermatology,* 2014. 31(4): p. 477-482.

[25] Castano, E., et al., Hypopigmented mycosis fungoides in childhood and adolescence: a long-term retrospective study. *Journal of cutaneous pathology,* 2013. 40(11): p. 924-934.

[26] Boccara, O., et al., Cutaneous hematologic disorders in children. *Pediatric blood & cancer,* 2012. 58(2): p. 226-232.

[27] Hodak, E., et al., Juvenile mycosis fungoides: cutaneous T-cell lymphoma with frequent follicular involvement. *Journal of the American Academy of Dermatology,* 2014. 70(6): p. 993-1001.

[28] Wohlmuth-Wieser, I., Primary cutaneous T-cell lymphomas in childhood and adolescence. *JDDG: Journal der Deutschen Dermatologischen Gesellschaft,* 2021. 19(4): p. 563-581.

[29] Tan, E.S.T., M.B.Y. Tang, and S.H. Tan, Retrospective 5-year review of 131 patients with mycosis fungoides and Sézary syndrome seen at the National Skin Centre, Singapore. *Australasian journal of dermatology,* 2006. 47(4): p. 248-252.

[30] Nasu-Tababuchi, M., et al., Hypopigmented mycosis fungoides: An immunological investigation of tumor-infiltrating T cells. *Dermatologica sinica,* 2016. 34(2): p. 96-98.

[31] Singh, Z.N., et al., Decreased CD117 expression in hypopigmented mycosis fungoides correlates with hypomelanosis: lessons learned from vitiligo. *Modern Pathology,* 2006. 19(9): p. 1255-1260.

[32] Rodney, I., et al., Hypopigmented mycosis fungoides: a retrospective clinicohistopathologic study. *Journal of the European Academy of Dermatology and Venereology,* 2017. 31(5): p. 808-814.

[33] Zang, J.B., et al., Pityriasis lichenoides: Long-term follow-up study. *Pediatric dermatology,* 2018. 35(2): p. 213-219.

[34] Bowers, S. and E.M. Warshaw, Pityriasis lichenoides and its subtypes. *Journal of the American Academy of Dermatology,* 2006. 55(4): p. 557-572.

[35] Khachemoune, A. and M.L. Blyumin, Pityriasis lichenoides. *American journal of clinical dermatology,* 2007. 8(1): p. 29-36.

[36] Geller, L., et al., Pityriasis lichenoides in childhood: review of clinical presentation and treatment options. *Pediatric dermatology,* 2015. 32(5): p. 579-592.

[37] Spergel, J.M. and A.S. Paller, Atopic dermatitis and the atopic march. *Journal of Allergy and Clinical Immunology,* 2003. 112(6): p. S118-S127.

[38] Kay, J., et al., The prevalence of childhood atopic eczema in a general population. *Journal of the American Academy of Dermatology,* 1994. 30(1): p. 35-39.

[39] Billings, S.D. and J. Cotton, *Spongiotic dermatitis, in Inflammatory Dermatopathology.* 2016, Springer. p. 5-21.

[40] Silverberg, N.B., Pediatric vitiligo. *Pediatric Clinics,* 2014. 61(2): p. 347-366.

[41] Handa, S. and S. Dogra, Epidemiology of childhood vitiligo: a study of 625 patients from north India. *Pediatric dermatology,* 2003. 20(3): p. 207-210.

[42] Hu, Z., et al., Profile of childhood vitiligo in China: an analysis of 541 patients. *Pediatric dermatology,* 2006. 23(2): p. 114-116.

[43] Halder, R.M., Childhood vitiligo. *Clinics in dermatology,* 1997. 15(6): p. 899-906. JAISHB; hydrogen bond forming ability.

[44] Ankar, T.J., M.C. Baruah, and B.R. Garg, Vitiligo in children. International journal of dermatology, 1992. 31(9): p. 621-623.

[45] Prcic, S., et al., Vitiligo in children. Pediatric dermatology, 2007. 24(6): p. 666-666.

[46] Kim, Y.C., et al., Histopathologic features in vitiligo. The American journal of dermatopathology, 2008. 30(2): p. 112-116.

[47] Bonifaz, A., et al., Tinea versicolor, tinea nigra, white piedra, and black piedra. Clinics in dermatology, 2010. 28(2): p. 140-145.

[48] Rios-Yuil, J.M., Pityriasis versicolor: clinical spectrum and diagnosis. Current Fungal Infection Reports, 2016. 10(3): p. 121-125.

[49] Zhou, H., et al., Dermoscopy as an ancillary tool for the diagnosis of pityriasis versicolor. Journal of the American Academy of Dermatology, 2015. 73(6): p. e205-e206.

[50] Hawkins, D.M. and A.C. Smidt, Superficial fungal infections in children. *Pediatric Clinics,* 2014. 61(2): p. 443-455.

[51] Miazek, N., et al., Pityriasis Alba—Common Disease, Enigmatic Entity: Up-to-Date Review of the Literature. *Pediatric dermatology,* 2015. 32(6): p. 786-791.

[52] Vachiramon, V. and K. Thadanipon, Postinflammatory hypopigmentation. *Clinical and Experimental Dermatology: Clinical dermatology,* 2011. 36(7): p. 708-714.

[53] Annessi, G., et al., Annular lichenoid dermatitis of youth. *Journal of the American Academy of Dermatology,* 2003. 49(6): p. 1029-1036.

[54] Kazlouskaya, V., J.D. Trager, and J.M. Junkins-Hopkins, Annular lichenoid dermatitis of youth: a separate entity or on the spectrum of mycosis fungoides? Case report and review of the literature. *Journal of cutaneous pathology,* 2015. 42(6): p. 420-426.

[55] Alikhan, A., et al., Pediatric follicular mucinosis: presentation, histopathology, molecular genetics, treatment, and outcomes over an 11-year period at the Mayo Clinic. *Pediatric dermatology,* 2013. 30(2): p. 192-198.

[56] Spence-Shishido, A., et al., Folliculotropic mycosis fungoides as a posttransplant lymphoproliferative disorder. Pediatrics, 2015. 136(3): p. e701-e705.

[57] Amitay-Laish, I., et al., Unilesional folliculotropic mycosis fungoides: a unique variant of cutaneous lymphoma. Journal of the European Academy of Dermatology and Venereology, 2016. 30(1): p. 25-29.

[58] Willemze, R., et al., WHO-EORTC classification for cutaneous lymphomas. Blood, 2005. 105(10): p. 3768-3785.

[59] Wang, D., et al., A review on pityriasis rubra pilaris. American journal of clinical dermatology, 2018. 19(3): p. 377-390.

[60] Klein, A., M. Landthaler, and S. Karrer, Pityriasis rubra pilaris. American journal of clinical dermatology, 2010. 11(3): p. 157-170.

[61] Ross, N.A., et al., Epidemiologic, clinicopathologic, diagnostic, and management challenges of pityriasis rubra pilaris: a case series of 100 patients. *JAMA dermatology,* 2016. 152(6): p. 670-675.

[62] Hwang, S. and R.A. Schwartz, Keratosis pilaris: a common follicular hyperkeratosis. *Cutis,* 2008. 82(3): p. 177-180.

[63] Poskitt, L. and J. Wilkinson, Natural history of keratosis pilaris. *British Journal of Dermatology,* 1994. 130(6): p. 711-713.

[64] Lehman, J.S., et al., Folliculotropic mycosis fungoides: single-center study and systematic review. *Archives of dermatology,* 2010. 146(6): p. 607-613.

[65] Zvulunov, A., et al., Clinical and histopathologic spectrum of alopecia mucinosa/follicular mucinosis and its natural history in children. *Journal of the American Academy of Dermatology,* 2012. 67(6): p. 1174-1181.

[66] Pimpinelli, N., et al., Defining early mycosis fungoides. Journal of the American Academy of Dermatology, 2005. 53(6): p. 1053-1063.

[67] Hodak, E. and I. Amitay-Laish, Mycosis fungoides: A great imitator. *Clinics in dermatology,* 2019. 37(3): p. 255-267.

[68] Pavlovsky, L., et al., Hyperpigmented mycosis fungoides: an unusual variant of cutaneous T-cell lymphoma with a frequent CD8+ phenotype. *Journal of the American Academy of Dermatology,* 2012. 67(1): p. 69-75.

[69] Virmani, P., et al., Clinical outcome and prognosis of young patients with mycosis fungoides. *Pediatric dermatology,* 2017. 34(5): p. 547-553.

[70] Tronnier, M., Foreign-body-associated granulomatous slack skin in folliculotropic mycosis fungoides of childhood. *Journal of cutaneous pathology,* 2009. 36(5): p. 578-581.

[71] Camacho, F.M., et al., Granulomatous slack skin in childhood. *Pediatric dermatology,* 1997. 14(3): p. 204-208.

[72] Moreno-Giménez, J., et al., Granulomatous slack skin disease in a child: the outcome. *Pediatric dermatology,* 2007. 24(6): p. 640-645.

[73] Wieser, I., C. Wohlmuth, and M. Duvic, Granulomatous mycosis fungoides in an adolescent—a rare encounter and review of the literature. *Pediatric dermatology,* 2016. 33(5): p. e296-e298.

[74] Lewis, D.J., et al., An adolescent with granulomatous mycosis fungoides infiltrating skeletal muscle successfully treated with oral prednisone. *JAAD case reports,* 2017. 3(4): p. 276.

[75] Tay, Y.K., W.L. Weston, and J.L. Aeling, Treatment of childhood cutaneous T-cell lymphoma with alpha-interferon plus PUVA. *Pediatric dermatology*, 1996. 13(6): p. 496-500.

[76] Wang, L., G. Wang, and T. Gao, Granulomatous syringotropic mycosis fungoides with two lesions having reactive B-cell proliferation. *Journal of cutaneous pathology,* 2014. 41(4): p. 400-406.

[77] Hazrati, L.N., V. Bril, and S. Nag, Muscle and nerve involvement in granulomatous mycosis fungoides. *Muscle & Nerve: Official Journal of the American Association of Electrodiagnostic Medicine,* 2007. 36(6): p. 860-865.

[78] Corbeddu, M., et al., Pagetoid reticulosis (Woringer-Kolopp disease) in a 2-year-old girl—Case report and review of the literature. *JAAD case reports,* 2019. 5(1): p. 104.

[79] Torre-Castro, J., et al., Pagetoid reticulosis in a 13-year old female. A unique immunohistochemical profile. *Journal of cutaneous pathology,* 2020. 47(5): p. 466-469.

[80] Mendese, G., et al., Pagetoid reticulosis in a prepubescent boy successfully treated with photodynamic therapy. *Clinical and Experimental Dermatology: Clinical dermatology,* 2012. 37(7): p. 759-761.

[81] Matsuzaki, Y., et al., Localized pagetoid reticulosis (Woringer-Kolopp disease) in early childhood. *Journal of the American Academy of Dermatology,* 2009. 61(1): p. 120-123.

[82] Miedler, J.D., et al., Pagetoid reticulosis in a 5-year-old boy. Journal of the American Academy of Dermatology, 2008. 58(4): p. 679-681.

[83] Evans, M.S., et al., Solitary plaque on the leg of a child: A report of two cases and a brief review of acral pseudolymphomatous angiokeratoma of children and unilesional mycosis fungoides. *Pediatric Dermatology,* 2019. 36(1): p. e1-e5.

[84] Kazakov, D., G. Burg, and W. Kempf, Clinicopathological spectrum of mycosis fungoides. *Journal of the European Academy of Dermatology and Venereology,* 2004. 18(4): p. 397-415.

[85] Rijlaarsdam, J.U., et al., Cutaneous pseudo-T-cell lymphomas. A clinicopathologic study of 20 patients. *Cancer,* 1992. 69(3): p. 717-24.

[86] Dippel, E., et al., S2k guidelines-cutaneous lymphomas update 2016-part 2: treatment and follow-up (ICD10 C82-C86). Journal der Deutschen Dermatologischen Gesellschaft. *Journal of the German Society of Dermatology:* JDDG, 2018. 16(1): p. 112-122.

[87] Guitart, J., et al., Histologic criteria for the diagnosis of mycosis fungoides: proposal for a grading system to standardize pathology reporting. *Journal of cutaneous pathology,* 2001. 28(4): p. 174-183.

[88] Kempf, W., et al., Granulomatous mycosis fungoides and granulomatous slack skin: a multicenter study of the Cutaneous Lymphoma Histopathology Task Force Group of the European Organization For Research and Treatment of Cancer (EORTC). *Archives of dermatology,* 2008. 144(12): p. 1609-1617.

[89] Haghighi, B., et al., Pagetoid reticulosis (Woringer-Kolopp disease): an immunophenotypic, molecular, and clinicopathologic study. *Modern Pathology,* 2000. 13(5): p. 502-510.

[90] Plaza, J.A., C. Morrison, and C.M. Magro, Assessment of TCR-β clonality in a diverse group of cutaneous T-Cell infiltrates. *Journal of cutaneous pathology,* 2008. 35(4): p. 358-365.

[91] Shiomi, T., et al., Poikilodermatous mycosis fungoides with a CD8+ CD56+ immunophenotype: a case report and literature review. *Journal of cutaneous pathology,* 2013. 40(3): p. 317-320.

[92] Poppe, H., et al., Childhood mycosis fungoides with a CD8+ CD56+ cytotoxic immunophenotype. *Journal of cutaneous pathology,* 2015. 42(4): p. 258-264.

[93] Ferenczi, K. and H.S. Makkar, Cutaneous lymphoma: Kids are not just little people. *Clinics in dermatology,* 2016. 34(6): p. 749-759.

[94] Gross, A.M., et al., A Pediatric Case of Transformed Mycosis Fungoides in a BRCA2 Positive Patient. *Journal of pediatric hematology/oncology,* 2020. 42(5): p. e361-e364.

[95] Alberti-Violetti, S., et al., Sézary Syndrome in a 17-Year-Old Boy: Clinicopathologic Features and Genomic Profile. *Pediatric dermatology,* 2016. 33(5): p. e318-e321.

[96] Meister, L., et al., Sézary syndrome in an 11-year-old girl. Journal of the American Academy of Dermatology, 1993. 28(1): p. 93-95.

[97] Molina, A., et al., Remission of refractory Sézary syndrome after bone marrow transplantation from a matched unrelated donor. *Biology of Blood and Marrow Transplantation,* 1999. 5(6): p. 400-404.

[98] Vermeer, M.H., et al., Novel and highly recurrent chromosomal alterations in Sézary syndrome. *Cancer research,* 2008. 68(8): p. 2689-2698.

[99] Caprini, E., et al., Identification of key regions and genes important in the pathogenesis of Sézary syndrome by combining genomic and expression microarrays. *Cancer research,* 2009. 69(21): p. 8438-8446.

[100] Espinet, B. and R. Salgado, Mycosis fungoides and Sézary syndrome, in *Array Comparative Genomic Hybridization.* 2013, Springer. p. 175-188.

[101] Salhany, K.E., et al., Transformation of cutaneous T cell lymphoma to large cell lymphoma. A clinicopathologic and immunologic study. *American Journal of Pathology,* 1988. 132(2): p. 265-77.

[102] Chan, W.H., et al., Juvenile mycosis fungoides with large-cell transformation: Successful treatment with psoralen with ultraviolet A light, interferon-alfa, and localized radiation. *Pediatric dermatology,* 2018. 35(1): p. e13-e16.

[103] Carrié, E., et al. Transformed juvenile-onset mycosis fungoides: treatment by bone marrow transplantation with graft-versus-lymphoma effect. In *Annales de Dermatologie et de Venereologie.* 2007.

[104] Romero, M., et al., Mycosis fungoides with focal CD 30 transformation in an adolescent. *Pediatric dermatology,* 2008. 25(5): p. 565-568.

[105] Pérez-Barrio, S., et al., Autologous hematopoietic stem cell transplantation followed by oral bexarotene in a patient with advanced

mycosis fungoides. *Actas Dermo-Sifiliográficas* (English Edition), 2008. 99(7): p. 560-564.

[106] Crowley, J.J., et al., Mycosis fungoides in young patients: clinical characteristics and outcome. *Journal of the American Academy of Dermatology,* 1998. 38(5): p. 696-701.

[107] Wieser, I., et al., Clinical characteristics, risk factors and long-term outcome of 114 patients with folliculotropic mycosis fungoides. *Archives of dermatological research,* 2017. 309(6): p. 453-459.

[108] Van Santen, S., et al., Clinical staging and prognostic factors in folliculotropic mycosis fungoides. *JAMA dermatology,* 2016. 152(9): p. 992-1000.

[109] Hodak, E., et al., New insights into folliculotropic mycosis fungoides (FMF): a single-center experience. *Journal of the American Academy of Dermatology,* 2016. 75(2): p. 347-355.

[110] Charli-Joseph, Y., et al., Association of a proposed new staging system for folliculotropic mycosis fungoides with prognostic variables in a US cohort. *JAMA dermatology,* 2021. 157(2): p. 157-165.

[111] Laggis, C.W., et al., Favourable outcomes in folliculotropic mycosis fungoides after multimodality treatment in a single institution. *Journal of the European Academy of Dermatology and Venereology,* 2021. 35(1): p. e42-e45.

[112] Gip, L. and E. Nilsson, Clustering of mycosis fungoides in the County of Västernorrland. *Lakartidningen,* 1977. 74(12): p. 1174-1176.

[113] Litvinov, I.V., et al., Identification of geographic clustering and regions spared by cutaneous T-cell lymphoma in Texas using 2 distinct cancer registries. *Cancer,* 2015. 121(12): p. 1993-2003.

[114] Moreau, J.F., et al., Non-random geographic distribution of patients with cutaneous T-cell lymphoma in the Greater Pittsburgh Area. *Dermatology Online Journal,* 2014. 20(7).

[115] Ghazawi, F.M., et al., Comprehensive analysis of cutaneous T-cell lymphoma (CTCL) incidence and mortality in Canada reveals changing trends and geographic clustering for this malignancy. *Cancer,* 2017. 123(18): p. 3550-3567.

[116] Ghazawi, F.M., et al., Environmental and other extrinsic risk factors contributing to the pathogenesis of cutaneous T cell lymphoma (CTCL). *Frontiers in oncology,* 2019. 9: p. 300.

[117] Fischmann, A., et al., Exposure to chemicals, physical agents, and biologic agents in mycosis fungoides and the Sézary syndrome. *Cancer treatment reports*, 1979. 63(4): p. 591-596.

[118] Chang, E.T. and E. Delzell, Systematic review and meta-analysis of glyphosate exposure and risk of lymphohematopoietic cancers. *Journal of Environmental Science and Health, Part B,* 2016. 51(6): p. 402-434.

[119] CAMERON, O.J., Mycosis fungoides in mother and in daughter. *Archives of Dermatology and Syphilology,* 1933. 27(2): p. 232-236.

[120] Sandbank, M. and I. Katzenellenbogen, Mycosis Fungoides of: Prolonged Duration in Siblings. *Archives of dermatology,* 1968. 98(6): p. 620-627.

[121] Cohen, S.R., et al., Mycosis fungoides: Clinicopathologic relationships, survival, and therapy in 59 patients with observations on occupation as a new prognostic factor. *Cancer,* 1980. 46(12): p. 2654-2666.

[122] Naji, A.A., M.M. Waiz, and K.E. Sharquie, Mycosis fungoides in identical twins. *Journal of the American Academy of Dermatology,* 2001. 44(3): p. 532-533.

[123] Hodak, E. and E. Friedman, Familial mycosis fungoides: model of genetic susceptibility. *Clinical Lymphoma, Myeloma and Leukemia,* 2010. 10: p. S67-S69.

[124] Hodak, E., et al., Familial mycosis fungoides: report of 6 kindreds and a study of the HLA system. *Journal of the American Academy of Dermatology,* 2005. 52(3): p. 393-402.

[125] Vassallo, C., et al., Mycosis fungoides in childhood: description and study of two siblings. *Acta dermato-venereologica,* 2007. 87(6): p. 529-532.

[126] Stern, R.S., K.T. Nichols, and L.H. Väkevä, Malignant melanoma in patients treated for psoriasis with methoxsalen (psoralen) and

ultraviolet A radiation (PUVA). *New England Journal of Medicine,* 1997. 336(15): p. 1041-1045.

[127] Juarez, M.C. and A.L. Grossberg, Phototherapy in the Pediatric Population. *Dermatologic clinics,* 2020. 38(1): p. 91-108.

[128] Moustafa, D., H. Neale, and E.B. Hawryluk, Trends in pediatric skin cancer. *Current Opinion in Pediatrics,* 2020. 32(4): p. 516-523.

[129] Hooper, M., et al., *Practice patterns in children, adolescents, and young adults with mycosis fungoides: Single institution study.* 2021, Wolters Kluwer Health.

[130] Lewis, D.J. and M. Duvic, Extracorporeal photopheresis for the treatment of early-stage mycosis fungoides. *Dermatologic therapy,* 2017. 30(3): p. e12485.

[131] Atilla, E., et al., Extracorporeal photochemotherapy in mycosis fungoides. *Transfusion clinique et biologique,* 2017. 24(4): p. 454-457.

In: Mycosis Fungoides and Sézary Syndrome ISBN: 978-1-68507-093-9
Editors: X. Zhang and L. Sokol

Chapter 8

Molecular Genetic Updates of Mycosis Fungoides

Hammad Tashkandi*, MD
Department of Pathology, H. Lee Moffitt Cancer Center and Research Institute, Tampa, FL, USA

Introduction

Mycosis fungoides (MF) is a T-cell lymphoproliferative disorder in which the neoplastic cells home the skin. Sézary syndrome (SS), on the other hand, is the leukemic variant with peripheral blood, skin, and lymph node involvement. MF/SS are recognized as separate entities but included in one staging system [1, 2]. Our understanding of the biology of MF/SS has been improved due to the remarkable advances in molecular studies.

Mycosis fungoides is routinely diagnosed by clinical and morphologic findings in the histologic and immunohistochemical studies of the atypical infiltrate. Molecular clonality assays can serve as diagnostic support, but few pathologists order them routinely based on a recent survey [3]. Further, few

* Corresponding Author's Email: hammad.tashkandi@moffitt.org.

pathologists rely on them for diagnosis for several reasons discussed in this chapter [3]. However, a subset of cases can be challenging and equivocal such as early lesions. Considering there is no definitive immunophenotypic marker for clonality in T-cells like the light chain restriction in B-cells, evaluating for clonality by molecular methods can help classify the lesions as benign or neoplastic, keeping in mind the caveats in interpreting these assays. Further, the clonality assays can be used to assess clonal relationships in multiple lesions.

Since MF is the most frequent form of cutaneous T-cell lymphomas (CTCLs) [2], it has been studied more extensively than other types of CTCLs. In recent years, high throughput sequencing studies with several reviews written revealed new insights into the biology of MF/SS. These findings offer prognostic information and novel targeted therapeutic strategies [4-7]. This chapter discusses the utility of molecular methods in diagnosis and the recent studies elucidating the genomic landscape of MF/SS.

Molecular Methods and Their Roles in Mycosis Fungoides

It is widely accepted that MF arises from a single clone of T-cells after acquiring oncogenic properties. The clonal property and the mutational profile can be utilized for diagnostic and prognostic purposes, as discussed below.

PCR and Sizing Based Assays

The rearrangement of T cell receptor (TCR) genes (*TRA, TRB, TRG, TRD*) that occur in the naïve T-cells in the thymus results in products with either heterodimer of alpha/beta or gamma/delta chains with unique rearrangements of their segments (V, D, and J). These rearrangements result in an enormous repertoire of T-cells. The addition and deletion of nucleotides can further expand this repertoire with the action of terminal deoxynucleotidyl transferase (TdT) enzyme at the junctions of the rearranged segments.

The rearrangement of the *TRG* gene generally occurs before *TRB*. The final developed T-cells contain rearranged *TRG* in both alpha/beta and gamma/delta T-cell types. Typically, for clonality assessment, both *TRG* and *TRB* loci are investigated. Some laboratories prefer testing for *TRG* gene rearrangement only as the *TRG* gene is rearranged first and is positive for clonal rearrangement in most T-cell neoplasms. Also, it has fewer segments, and therefore fewer primers are required for PCR amplification [8]. However, combined testing with the *TRB* gene primers increases the sensitivity [9, 10].

The unique rearrangements result in different lengths of DNA segments, which can be targeted using universal primers for diagnostic purposes (Fig. 8-1). PCR amplification of products of the same size, which various methods can visualize, indicates clonality in straightforward cases (Fig. 8-2) [11, 12]. Capillary gel electrophoresis is more sensitive than conventional polyacrylamide gel analysis in visualizing the PCR products and has a semiquantitative advantage [13, 14]. The choice of oligonucleotide primers and PCR design markedly impact the success of PCR-based assays in clonality assessment. However, using a standardized set of primers, e.g., BIOMED 2, could increase the diagnostic yield and standardize the process [9, 15, 16].

A normal population of T-cells would typically show a polyclonal pattern in the sizing assay (Fig. 8-2). In contrast, clonal results show one or two clonal peaks based on the number of rearranged alleles and primer set design. The PCR products typically have a size range for expected polyclonal and clonal peaks. Peaks located outside of the range may result from non-specific PCR amplification. However, true clonal results may appear outside the range due to amplification of downstream segments or partial deletion of segments [17]. If such cases are suspected, TCR clonality assessment by sequencing the TCR gene might confirm the clonality. Of note, many neoplastic cases do not have a dominant clone, while a dominant peak may represent a mixture of clones of similar size [18]. Therefore, it is recommended to run the PCR in duplicate, and only reproducible peaks should be considered positive [8]. Further, some malignancies fail to show a clonal pattern for various technical reasons. Therefore, the monoclonal result should be interpreted in the appropriate morphologic and clinical setting.

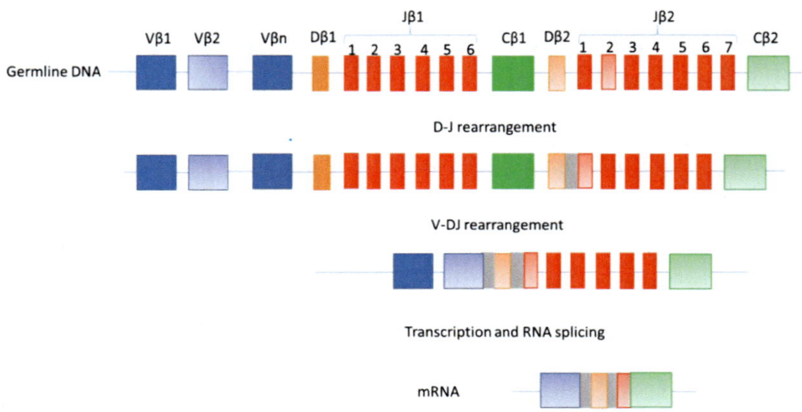

Figure 8-1. An example of the TRB gene illustrating the rearrangement of the variable (V), diversity (D), joining (J), and constant (C) segments. The gradient color boxes represent the selected segments in the final rearranged products. The light grey box represents changes in the germline sequence due to nucleotide addition and deletions. Depending on the selected segments, the sizes of the DNA segments vary in different T-cells, which is the principle used in the sizing assays by PCR.

The limit of detection depends on various factors, including assay designs, the degree of polyclonal background, and detection methods. The widely used BIOMED-2 primer sets are reported to have a limit of detection of 1-10% clonal cells [16]. The clinical sensitivity of detecting clonality by PCR is variable in different studies, and ranging from 50–90% [19-21]. False-negative results can be due to various reasons such as interobserver variability between molecular pathologists, insufficient tumor cells or primer designs that fail to anneal to the target locus, or lack of primers that target a particular segment of the gene. As an example of the latter, in BIOMED-2 primer sets, there is no primer for Jγ1.2 (JγP) [16]. This segment is used in the rearrangement in about 3% of T-cell neoplasms [22]. In rare cases, where only one allele with Jγ1.2 is rearranged, the result may be falsely negative. Despite the variable clinical sensitivities, monoclonal results can be used as an adjunct to confirm or reclassify some cases with additional clinical and pathologic findings [15, 23].

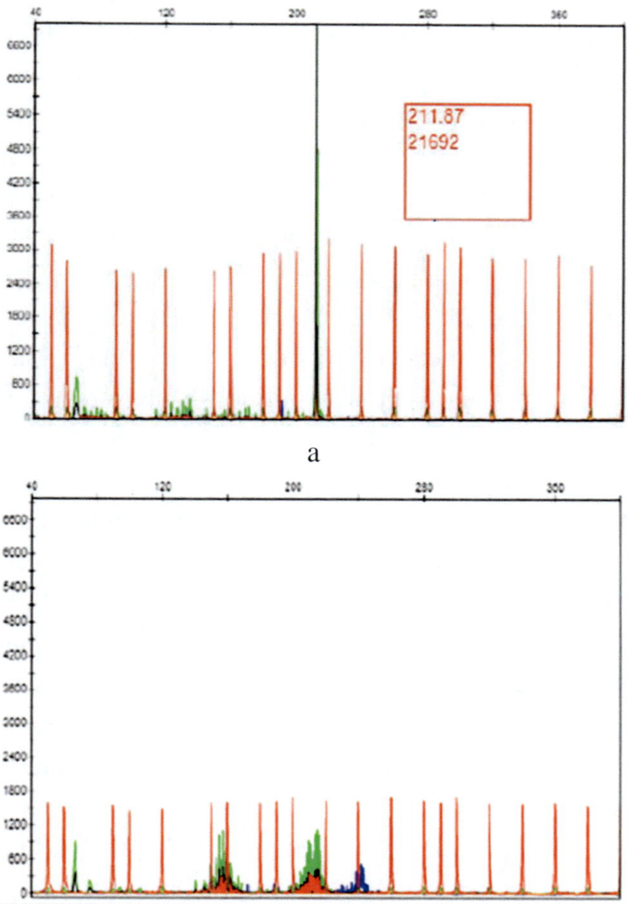

a

b

Figure 8-2. Examples of capillary electropherograms for TRG gene analysis by BIOMED-2 primer sets. The assays show clonal result (A) and polyclonal result (B). The X-axis represents the amplitude height, and it correlates with the extent of the clone, while the Y-axis represents the approximate number of nucleotides in the PCR product.

The lack of specificity of clonal T-cells is a diagnostic limitation. Clonal T-cells have been reported in non-neoplastic conditions such as autoimmune disorders, viral infections, and reactive lymphoid proliferations [24]. True cross lineage T-cell gene rearrangements have been reported in mature B-cell neoplasms, and in approximately 10% of cases, strong clonal patterns were detected, suggesting true cross lineage rearrangements [25]. Further, many benign inflammatory dermatoses, including lichen planus, pityriasis lichenoides, lichen sclerosus, granuloma annulare and chronic eczema, and benign lymphoproliferative disorders such as lymphomatoid papulosis (LyP), can be associated with clonal T-cells[26-33]. In one study, over 40% of LyP were associated with clonally rearranged T-cells [34]. The specificity of clonality testing by PCR can be improved by identifying identical clones in two different sites [21, 35]. Comparing the clonal peaks identified in different samples is especially useful in cases where the polyclonal background obscures the malignant clone in PCR analysis, as long as distinct peaks are present. Additionally, identifying identical clonal peaks in different anatomic sites was more likely to be associated with progressive disease than clonal heterogeneity, in which clonal peaks are different in different anatomic sites, as has been reported in 30-48% of MF [21, 36].

A limited lymphocyte repertoire can potentially confound the interpretation leading to pseudoclonality [8]. Duplicate testing may show different size peaks, confirming pseudoclonality. Sometimes, oligoclonal proliferation can be detected with the presence of more than two clonal peaks. An oligoclonal pattern can be seen in situations with restricted T-cell repertoire, seen in older individuals and during immune reconstitution after chemotherapy or stem cell transplantation [37-39]. In these instances, if there is an amplification bias of the PCR products, the result may appear clonal. Moreover, testing the peripheral blood of patients with MF may seem clonal. However, the sizes of the peaks are usually different from those detected in the skin, indicating non-neoplastic clone and pseudoclonality.

In addition to the previous biologic causes of clonal T-cells, the interpretation of clonality assays could be prone to interobserver variability and potentially false positive results. However, applying more stringent interpretative criteria can improve the specificity of the test [40].

Nonetheless, using specific cut-off for interpretation may create a false sense of accuracy and false-positive and negative results, as these tests are qualitative rather than quantitative. Currently, there are no universally applied criteria for interpretation. Therefore, each laboratory should establish interpretative standards for their assays, considering the caveats discussed here [12].

In MF/SS, PCR-based clonality assays can be used for monitoring residual disease by following up the clonal peak(s) initially identified [1]. However, this assessment is not suitable for minimal residual disease (MRD) monitoring as the clonal peak can be hard to distinguish from a polyclonal background. Further, evaluation of residual disease by PCR-based method did not show a significant prognostic difference [41, 42]. However, assessment for MRD by sequencing methods provides much deeper sensitivity and may provide prognostic information (see below).

Next Generation Sequencing Based Assays

Next generation sequencing (NGS) based assays can be used for molecular profiling and clonality assessment. Molecular profiling using NGS technology allows for detecting single nucleotide variants, copy number alterations, chromosomal translocations, and even gene expression levels. The sequencing can be performed on both DNA and RNA and customized to a selected number of genes based on clinical needs. The molecular profiles of MF/SS using NGS will be discussed below (see Molecular profiles of Mycosis fungoides/sézary syndrome and their prognostic significance and role in targeted therapies).

NGS has a much higher clinical sensitivity than PCR-based clonality assays [18, 43-45]. In an NGS-based assay, the PCR products are ligated into adaptors in a single chip and parallelly sequenced. The neoplastic clone is identified by sequence frequency rather than relying on the amplitude height of a PCR product with a specific size, which can be obscured when polyclonal PCR products are present [44]. Further, it has a higher specificity than PCR in distinguishing neoplastic from benign lesions [18, 43]. The limit of detection can be as low as 1 in 50,000 cells. Therefore, it is more reliable in identifying MRD [43, 46].

Monitoring for MRD by NGS has become increasingly important for clinical decision-making in various hematopoietic neoplasms, including acute lymphocytic leukemia and multiple myeloma [47, 48]. However, similar prognostic studies have not been implemented in MF/SS. Weng et al. showed that MRD detection by this method is highly sensitive and specific [46]. A more recent study demonstrated that when compared to flow cytometry and conventional PCR analysis, detection of the clonal sequence in peripheral blood has the highest specificity [49]. However, the impact of MRD positivity post therapy on outcome and prognosis is yet unclear.

Moreover, NGS-based assays have the advantage of being quantitative. In a study evaluating the use of NGS in predicting prognosis in MF, the tumor clone frequency (TCF) was an independent prognostic marker for progression-free and overall survival. In early MF, more than 25% of TCF was a strong predictive marker of progression than any other established prognostic markers [50]. Early identification of patients at higher risk of progression may help guide therapeutic decisions.

Gene Expression Profiling

Several methods are available for RNA profiling using reverse transcriptase (RT)-PCR technology. Whole transcriptome analysis using RNAseq can be performed, or more practically, panels of selected genes can be designed and validated for clinical use [51]. Although several of these methods require testing fresh samples as the RNA is relatively unstable, newer clinically validated assays can be performed on formalin-fixed paraffin-embedded tissue (FFPE) [52, 53].

Several studies showed that gene expression profiling could differentiate benign inflammatory dermatosis from MF and provide prognostic information that cannot be gleaned from histologic and clinical findings alone, especially in early MF. Some studies investigated different gene expression diagnostic assays for MF/SS, and they showed high clinical sensitivity reaching or approaching 100% even with a limited panel of 4 genes [54-56]. Notably, *TOX* gene is upregulated in early MF and can help identify patients at risk of progression and differentiate MF from benign dermatoses [54, 57]. Furthermore, high expression of *TOX* is strongly correlated with disease progression [58].

Moreover, gene expression profiling can be used to identify therapeutic targets. *CD158k/KIR3DL2* is highly expressed in advanced MF and can be targeted using monoclonal antibody agents [59, 60]. Also, the expression of *CCR4* can be detected by gene expression profiling. MF with high expression of *CCR4* could be targeted by anti-CCR4 monoclonal antibody mogamulizumab, which the FDA has approved to treat refractory MF and SS [61].

MicroRNA Profiling

MicroRNAs are short non-coding RNA with an average length of 22 nucleotides. They are involved in regulating gene expression [62]. Early MF and benign lesions display different microRNAs profiles. Moreover, microRNAs are deregulated as the disease progresses to an advanced stage [63]. Similar to gene expression profiling, microRNA profiling has been evaluated for diagnostic purposes in MF/SS. A limited panel of three microRNAs (miR-155, miR-203, and miR-205) have been investigated, and it revealed 95% sensitivity and specificity in distinguishing early MF from benign lesions [64]. Moreover, monitoring their levels in plasma can be used to assess response to therapy [65]. Another 3-miRNA classifier (miR-106b-5p, miR-148a-3p, and miR-338-3p) has been studied, and it successfully classified patients into high-risk and low-risk groups of disease progression [66].

Single Cell Sequencing

Single-cell sequencing of RNA allows sequencing of thousands of cells in one sample and, therefore, can demonstrate the constituents of the microenvironment, tumor heterogeneity, and potential mechanisms for drug resistance. Although it is mainly used for research purposes, few studies showed its potential role in precision medicine, setting the ground for its use in the coming years for routine clinical care, at least in refractory cases [67, 68]. Several studies show that single-cell RNA sequencing revealed high inter-tumor and intra-tumor heterogeneity in MF [69-71]. Interestingly, Buus et al. demonstrated that a subpopulation of tumor cells in SS was resistant to treatment while others were responsive. The findings provide a potential mechanism for disease progression and relapse while on therapy [70].

Molecular Profiles of Mycosis Fungoides/Sézary Syndrome and Their Prognostic Significance and Role in Targeted Therapies

Molecular abnormalities in MF/SS are heterogeneous and not specific. However, some alterations can be seen more frequently than others. Whole-exome/genome NGS and array comparative genomic hybridization studies revealed several alterations in various pathways that drive oncogenesis, providing potential prognostic information and therapeutic targets. These pathways include the cell cycle and DNA damage repair, JAK-STAT signaling, TCR/NF-κB signaling, chromatin-modifying genes, and MAPK pathway [72, 73].

The molecular profiling shows that most MF/SS cases are driven by copy number alterations (CNA) rather than single nucleotide variation. CNA comprise approximately 40- 92% of the mutations [72, 74-76]. The higher frequency of CNA could be in part explained by the aberrantly activated recombinase activating gene (RAG) endonucleases in MF, which are generally involved in the recombination events in normal T-cells [74]. Interestingly, sequencing studies show a high frequency of transitional mutations (C to T). These alterations are detected in 40–60% of cases and may suggest that ultraviolet B exposure of the skin-homing T-lymphocytes may contribute to the pathogenesis of MF [73, 77]. The various pathways affected in MF/SS and potential therapeutic targeting will be discussed in this section (Table 8-1).

Table 8-1. Altered molecular pathways and potential therapeutic considerations in MF/SS

Signaling pathways/genes	Prevalence of alteration (CNV/mutation)	Potential targeted therapies
Cell cycle regulators		
CDKN1B	15%	CDK inhibitor
CDKN2A	60%	
RB1	25%	
TP53	30%	Resistance to MDM2 Inhibitor
RPS6KA1	36%	
ATR	6%	
MYC	40%	BET inhibitor
JAK-STAT signaling		
JAK1	3%	JAK inhibitor
JAK3	4%	JAK inhibitor
STAT3	3%	
STAT5B	3%	
MAPK signaling		
KRAS	<1%	
NRAS	<1%	
BRAF	<1%	
MAP2K1	<1%	
MAPK1	<1%	
TCR/NF-κB signaling		
PLCG1	15%	Calcineurin inhibitor
PTEN	20%	PI3K inhibitor, mTOR inhibitor
RhoA	6%	
PRKG	6%	
PRKCQ	30%	
CARD11	12%	Proteasome inhibitor
TNFAIP3	22%	
NFKB2	6%	Proteasome inhibitor resistance
PDCD1	35%	

Table 8-1. (Continued)

Signaling pathways/genes	Prevalence of alteration (CNV/mutation)	Potential targeted therapies
TCR/NF-κB signaling		
CD28	12%	Anti-CD80/CD86
CD28-CTLA4, CD28-ICOS	4%	Anti-CTLA4
Notch	100% (n=5)	GSI
TNFRSF1B (TNFR2)	6%	Proteasome inhibitor
TNFRSF6	10%	
CCR4	7%	Mogamulizumab (Anti-CCR4)
ZEB1	43%	
DNA methylation		
DNMT3A	18%	Hypomethylating agents
DNMT3B	11%	
TET1	10%	
TET2	10%	
Histone methylation and acetylation		
MLL2	10%	
MLL3	60%	
MLL4	18%	
SETD1A	16%	
SETD1B	16%	
SETDB2	22%	
SETD6	11%	
KDM6B	50%	
CREBBP	5%	
NCOR1	50%	HDAC inhibitors
Chromatin remodeling		
ARID1A	20%	
ARID5B	29%	
SMARCC1	21%	
ARID1B, ARID4A	< 10%	
ARID2	< 10%	
ARID3A	< 10%	
SMARCA4	< 10%	
CHD3	< 10%	

Adapted and modified from Elenitoba-Johnson et al. [7].

Cell Cycle Regulators

CNA in cell cycle regulators are frequent in MF/SS. Deletions of *CDKN1A* (11%) and *CDKN2A* (40%) have been reported, along with deletions of *ATM* (30%), *RB1* (39%), and *TP53* (93%) [74, 77]. *TP53* mutations and *CDKN2A* deletions were significantly enriched in patients with large cell transformation [77]. These findings need further validation in larger studies to confirm the prognostic significance. In one study, MYC showed a gain in 40% of SS cases, suggesting it has an oncogenic role in stimulating cell cycle progression [78].

JAK-STAT Signaling

Activating point mutations in JAK/STAT pathway are reported in *JAK1* (0.9%), *JAK3* (2.7%), *STAT3* (0.9%), and *STAT5B* (3.6%). Besides, copy number gains of *JAK2* (13%), *STAT3* (60%), and *STAT5B* (60%) are reported and show a correlation with increased expression of these genes [79]. Moreover, *HNRNPK* and *SOCS1*, which are inhibitors of JAK-STAT signaling, are recurrently deleted in MF. Currently, there are FDA-approved JAK inhibitors such as tofacitinib and ruxolitinib. These drugs have been tested in vivo with promising results [72-74, 80].

MAPK Signaling

A relatively small subset of SS/MF patients have activating mutations in the pathway (<1%), including a gain of function mutations in *KRAS, NRAS, BRAF, MAP2K1*, and *MAPK1* [79]. Although these mutations are relatively infrequent in MF/SS, several studies and clinical trials in solid tumor malignancies show that these mutations can be druggable with promising results [81-83]. The findings may provide hope in a subset of cases with these alterations.

TCR/NF-κB Signaling

Not surprisingly, mutations in various elements of the TCR pathway in SS/MF are frequent and result in augmented signaling [72, 74, 75, 77]. Point mutations in *CD28* (3.6% of cases) increase its affinity for B7 ligands (CD80 and CD86) and subsequently result in increased TCR signaling. Similarly, *CD28-ICOS* and *CD28-CTLA4* gene fusions are reported in few patients with MF/SS and result in activation of TCR signaling [75, 77, 79, 84]. Immunotherapy with anti-CTLA4 has been tested against tumors with *CD28-CTLA4* gene fusion with promising results [84]. Point mutations (10% of cases) and copy number gains (5%) in *PLCG1* eventually enhance antigen-dependent T-cell activation [79, 85]. Furthermore, point mutations in *PRKCB* and *PRKCQ* (<1% of cases) and amplification of the latter (30%) may contribute to TCR signaling deregulation [79]. Also, inactivating point mutations and deletions in *ZEB1* (56–65%) lead to overproduction of TH2 cytokines promoting tumor growth [73, 74, 77].

TCR activation subsequently activates NF-κB signaling through the canonical pathway. Point mutations (5.4% of cases) and copy number gains (23%) in SS/MF involving *CARD11* lead to increased NF-κB activation [72, 75, 79]. The latter alteration has been suggested as a potential therapeutic target [74]. In addition, recurrent deletions of *NFKB2* (2.5% of cases) are predicted to cause proteasomal IkB cleavage and constitutively activate the pathway [74, 75, 79]. These alterations could potentially be targeted by proteasome inhibitors [86]. Furthermore, receptors other than the TCR complex can also activate canonical NF-κB signaling. Point mutations (2.2%) and amplifications (2.5%) in *TNFRSF1B* have been reported to constitutively activate NF-κB signaling [75, 79]. In one study, 18% of patients with MF/SS had *TNFRSF1B* alterations, including copy number gain and a recurrent gain of function mutation (Thr377Ile) identified in 5% of cases [75]. Similarly, *TNFAIP3*, an inhibitor in NF-κB signaling, was deleted in 25% of SS cases [79].

In vitro studies inhibiting the NF-κB pathway through proteasome inhibitors showed increased apoptosis of SS cells [87, 88]. Moreover, in a phase II study assessing a proteasome inhibitor (bortezomib) in MF patients, the toxicity was relatively limited. The overall response rate for MF was 67%, and the complete response rate was 17% [89]. These findings indicate that targeting the NF-κB pathway could be a potential therapy, at least in combination with other drugs.

DNA Methylation

Mutational profiling shows that widespread changes in DNA methylation characterize MF/SS, in part due to mutations in genes coding for DNA methylation enzymes [90]. Loss of function alterations in DNA methyltransferases such as *DNMT3A* through deletion are frequently reported in SS (38%). Besides, mutations are reported in a subset of cases (4%). These alterations can lead to global hypomethylation. In contrast, fewer inactivating alterations in demethylating proteins such as *TET2* are reported in MF/SS. *TET2* mutations and deletions are reported in 3.6% and 2.5% of SS cases, respectively. Mutations in genes coding histone demethylases, such as *KMT2C*, *KMT2D*, and *KDM6A*, are reported in 2.2%, 3.1%, and 1.3% of MF/SS cases, respectively. However, *SETDB2*, another gene encoding for histone demethylase enzyme, is deleted in 28% of MF/SS patients [79]. Overall, the methylation profile of MF/SS suggests that demethylating agents could be a potential therapeutic option.

Histone Methylation and Acetylation

Deletions and point mutations in genes involving histone acetyltransferase such as *CREBBP* are relatively infrequent in MF/SS and reported in 3.1% and 2.5% of cases, respectively. An adapter protein TRRAP, with histone acetyltransferase activity, is amplified in 10% of patients and mutated in 4.9% of cases [79]. Moreover, point mutations in gene encoding histone deacetylases such as *NCOR1* and *BCOR* are infrequent and reported in 3.1% and 2.7% of the MF/SS cases, respectively [79]. However, deletions in genes encoding histone deacetylases such as *NCOR1* are frequent and reported in 80% of MF/SS patients [79]. Of note, two HDAC inhibitors (romidepsin and vorinostat) are currently FDA approved for MF treatment [1].

Chromatin Remodeling

Deletions of genes involved in chromatin remodeling are relatively frequent in SS, and deletions of *ARID1A* (58%), *ARID5B* (29%), and *SMARCC1* (21%) are the most frequent alterations [79, 91]. In contrast, point mutations in *ARID2* and *SMARCB1* are less frequent and reported in a subset of MF/SS cases [73].

Chromothripsis

Chromothripsis represents catastrophic cellular events that result in tens to hundreds of rearrangements occurring in few chromosomal loci [92]. Chromothripsis is observed in higher frequency in MF than other cancers and reported in up to 65% of cases. The catastrophic events most often involve chromosomes 10, 2, and 1, in descending order of frequency. These events impact several tumor suppressor genes and may explain the frequent deletions of these genes in MF/SS [74].

CONCLUSION

The advancement of molecular techniques has markedly improved our understanding of MF/SS. Whole-genome studies showed that MF/SS are genetically complex. Nevertheless, molecular studies reveal genetically distinct molecular profiles characterized by frequent CNA and transitional mutations. Many of these alterations could be targeted, particularly in refractory cases.

Besides the conventional clonality assays, molecular assays could help diagnose early and equivocal cases using NGS and gene expression studies analyzing CNA, single nucleotide variants, and gene expression levels. Comparable assays are currently clinically validated for solid tumor confirmation in single panels such as Thyroseq and Pancreaseq [93, 94].

Similar assays could be developed to confirm the diagnoses in challenging cases of MF.

In addition to confirming the diagnosis, molecular profiling enables prognostication and establishing therapeutic targets. The prior studies were performed on relatively small cohorts. The prognostic implications of genetic findings need to be validated, which is only possible with more frequent molecular profiling for cases. Further, assessment for MRD by NGS may facilitate evaluation for response to therapy and monitoring for the residual disease at a deeper level. It may guide therapeutic decisions similar to MRD assessment in other hematopoietic neoplasms.

References

[1] Olsen, E., et al., Revisions to the staging and classification of mycosis fungoides and Sézary syndrome: a proposal of the International Society for Cutaneous Lymphomas (ISCL) and the cutaneous lymphoma task force of the European Organization of Research and Treatment of Cancer (EORTC). *Blood,* 2007. 110(6): p. 1713-22.

[2] Willemze, R., et al., The 2018 update of the WHO-EORTC classification for primary cutaneous lymphomas. *Blood,* 2019. 133(16): p. 1703-1714.

[3] Comfere, N., et al., Views of dermatopathologists about clonality assays in the diagnosis of cutaneous T-cell and B-cell lymphoproliferative disorders. *J Cutan Pathol,* 2018. 45(1): p. 39-47.

[4] Walia, R. and C.C.S. Yeung, An Update on Molecular Biology of Cutaneous T Cell Lymphoma. *Front Oncol,* 2019. 9: p. 1558.

[5] Bastidas Torres, A. N., et al., Molecular advances in cutaneous T-cell lymphoma. *Semin Cutan Med Surg,* 2018. 37(1): p. 81-86.

[6] Larocca, C. and T. Kupper, Mycosis Fungoides and Sézary Syndrome: An Update. *Hematol Oncol Clin North Am,* 2019. 33(1): p. 103-120.

[7] Elenitoba-Johnson, K. S. and R. Wilcox, A new molecular paradigm in mycosis fungoides and Sézary syndrome. *Semin Diagn Pathol,* 2017. 34(1): p. 15-21.

[8] Raess, P. W. and A. Bagg, The role of molecular pathology in the diagnosis of cutaneous lymphomas. *Patholog Res Int,* 2012. 2012(913523): p. 913523.
[9] Lukowsky, A., et al., Evaluation of T-cell clonality in archival skin biopsy samples of cutaneous T-cell lymphomas using the biomed-2 PCR protocol. *Diagn Mol Pathol,* 2010. 19(2): p. 70-7.
[10] Zhang, B., et al., Combined use of PCR-based TCRG and TCRB clonality tests on paraffin-embedded skin tissue in the differential diagnosis of mycosis fungoides and inflammatory dermatoses. *J Mol Diagn,* 2010. 12(3): p. 320-7.
[11] Wood, G. S., Analysis of clonality in cutaneous T cell lymphoma and associated diseases. *Ann N Y Acad Sci,* 2001. 941(1): p. 26-30.
[12] Langerak, A. W., et al., EuroClonality/BIOMED-2 guidelines for interpretation and reporting of Ig/TCR clonality testing in suspected lymphoproliferations. *Leukemia,* 2012. 26(10): p. 2159-71.
[13] Lee, S. C., et al., Pseudo-spikes are common in histologically benign lymphoid tissues. *J Mol Diagn,* 2000. 2(3): p. 145-52.
[14] Tang, M. B., et al., A comparative study of polymerase chain reaction detection of clonal T-cell receptor gamma chain gene rearrangements using polyacrylamide gel electrophoresis versus fluorescence capillary electrophoresis. *Ann Acad Med Singap,* 2008. 37(1): p. 27-31.
[15] Sandberg, Y., et al., Molecular immunoglobulin/T- cell receptor clonality analysis in cutaneous lymphoproliferations. Experience with the BIOMED-2 standardized polymerase chain reaction protocol. *Haematologica*, 2003. 88(6): p. 659-70.
[16] van Dongen, J. J., et al., Design and standardization of PCR primers and protocols for detection of clonal immunoglobulin and T-cell receptor gene recombinations in suspect lymphoproliferations: report of the BIOMED-2 Concerted Action BMH4-CT98-3936. *Leukemia,* 2003. 17(12): p. 2257-317.
[17] Langerak, A. W., Undersized, oversized? It is not one-size-fits-all in lymphoid clonality detection. *Leuk Res,* 2008. 32(2): p. 203-4.
[18] Schumacher, J. A., et al., A comparison of deep sequencing of TCRG rearrangements vs traditional capillary electrophoresis for assessment

of clonality in T-Cell lymphoproliferative disorders. *Am J Clin Pathol,* 2014. 141(3): p. 348-59.

[19] Hodges, E., et al., Diagnostic role of tests for T cell receptor (TCR) genes. *J Clin Pathol,* 2003. 56(1): p. 1-11.

[20] Hsiao, P. F., et al., Histopathologic-molecular correlation in early mycosis fungoides using T-cell receptor gamma gene rearrangement by polymerase chain reaction with laser capture microdissection. *J Formos Med Assoc,* 2007. 106(4): p. 265-72.

[21] Ponti, R., et al., TCRgamma-chain gene rearrangement by PCR-based GeneScan: diagnostic accuracy improvement and clonal heterogeneity analysis in multiple cutaneous T-cell lymphoma samples. *J Invest Dermatol,* 2008. 128(4): p. 1030-8.

[22] Lawnicki, L.C., et al., The distribution of gene segments in T-cell receptor gamma gene rearrangements demonstrates the need for multiple primer sets. *J Mol Diagn,* 2003. 5(2): p. 82-7.

[23] Alessi, E., et al., The usefulness of clonality for the detection of cases clinically and/or histopathologically not recognized as cutaneous T-cell lymphoma. *Br J Dermatol,* 2005. 153(2): p. 368-71.

[24] Langerak, A. W., et al., Polymerase chain reaction-based clonality testing in tissue samples with reactive lymphoproliferations: usefulness and pitfalls. A report of the BIOMED-2 Concerted Action BMH4-CT98-3936. *Leukemia,* 2007. 21(2): p. 222-9.

[25] Evans, P. A., et al., Significantly improved PCR-based clonality testing in B-cell malignancies by use of multiple immunoglobulin gene targets. Report of the BIOMED-2 Concerted Action BHM4-CT98-3936. *Leukemia,* 2007. 21(2): p. 207-14.

[26] Pfaltz, K., et al., Clonality in sarcoidosis, granuloma annulare, and granulomatous mycosis fungoides. *Am J Dermatopathol,* 2011. 33(7): p. 659-62.

[27] Dippel, E., et al., Clonal T-cell receptor gamma-chain gene rearrangement by PCR-based GeneScan analysis in advanced cutaneous T-cell lymphoma: a critical evaluation. *J Pathol,* 1999. 188(2): p. 146-54.

[28] Jawed, S. I., et al., Primary cutaneous T-cell lymphoma (mycosis fungoides and Sézary syndrome): part I. Diagnosis: clinical and histopathologic features and new molecular and biologic markers. *J Am Acad Dermatol,* 2014. 70(2): p. 205 e1-16; quiz 221-2.

[29] Ponti, R., et al., T-cell receptor gamma gene rearrangement by multiplex polymerase chain reaction/heteroduplex analysis in patients with cutaneous T-cell lymphoma (mycosis fungoides/Sézary syndrome) and benign inflammatory disease: correlation with clinical, histological and immunophenotypical findings. *Br J Dermatol,* 2005. 153(3): p. 565-73.

[30] Lukowsky, A., et al., Detection of expanded T cell clones in skin biopsy samples of patients with lichen sclerosus et atrophicus by T cell receptor-gamma polymerase chain reaction assays. *J Invest Dermatol,* 2000. 115(2): p. 254-9.

[31] Schiller, P. I., et al., Detection of clonal T cells in lichen planus. *Arch Dermatol Res,* 2000. 292(11): p. 568-9.

[32] Shieh, S., D. L. Mikkola, and G. S. Wood, Differentiation and clonality of lesional lymphocytes in pityriasis lichenoides chronica. *Arch Dermatol,* 2001. 137(3): p. 305-8.

[33] Dereure, O., E. Levi, and M. E. Kadin, T-Cell clonality in pityriasis lichenoides et varioliformis acuta: a heteroduplex analysis of 20 cases. *Arch Dermatol,* 2000. 136(12): p. 1483-6.

[34] el-Azhary, R. A., et al., Lymphomatoid papulosis: a clinical and histopathologic review of 53 cases with leukocyte immunophenotyping, DNA flow cytometry, and T-cell receptor gene rearrangement studies. *J Am Acad Dermatol,* 1994. 30(2 Pt 1): p. 210-8.

[35] Thurber, S. E., et al., T-cell clonality analysis in biopsy specimens from two different skin sites shows high specificity in the diagnosis of patients with suggested mycosis fungoides. *J Am Acad Dermatol,* 2007. 57(5): p. 782-90.

[36] Vega, F., et al., Clonal heterogeneity in mycosis fungoides and its relationship to clinical course. *Blood,* 2002. 100(9): p. 3369-73.

[37] Sarzotti, M., et al., T cell repertoire development in humans with SCID after nonablative allogeneic marrow transplantation. *J Immunol,* 2003. 170(5): p. 2711-8.

[38] Mariani, S., et al., Severe and long-lasting disruption of T-cell receptor diversity in human myeloma after high-dose chemotherapy and autologous peripheral blood progenitor cell infusion. *Br J Haematol,* 2001. 113(4): p. 1051-9.

[39] Delfau-Larue, M. H., et al., Diagnostic value of dominant T-cell clones in peripheral blood in 363 patients presenting consecutively with a clinical suspicion of cutaneous lymphoma. *Blood,* 2000. 96(9): p. 2987-92.

[40] Cushman-Vokoun, A. M., S. Connealy, and T. C. Greiner, Assay design affects the interpretation of T-cell receptor gamma gene rearrangements: comparison of the performance of a one-tube assay with the BIOMED-2-based TCRG gene clonality assay. *J Mol Diagn,* 2010. 12(6): p. 787-96.

[41] Hurabielle, C., et al., Frequency and prognostic value of cutaneous molecular residual disease in mycosis fungoides: a prospective multicentre trial of the Cutaneous Lymphoma French Study Group. *Br J Dermatol,* 2015. 173(4): p. 1015-23.

[42] Massone, C., et al., The prognosis of early mycosis fungoides is not influenced by phenotype and T-cell clonality. *Br J Dermatol,* 2008. 159(4): p. 881-6.

[43] Kirsch, I. R., et al., TCR sequencing facilitates diagnosis and identifies mature T cells as the cell of origin in CTCL. *Sci Transl Med,* 2015. 7(308): p. 308ra158.

[44] Sufficool, K. E., et al., T-cell clonality assessment by next-generation sequencing improves detection sensitivity in mycosis fungoides. *J Am Acad Dermatol,* 2015. 73(2): p. 228-36 e2.

[45] Rea, B., et al., Role of high-throughput sequencing in the diagnosis of cutaneous T-cell lymphoma. *J Clin Pathol,* 2018. 71(9): p. 814-820.

[46] Weng, W. K., et al., Minimal residual disease monitoring with high-throughput sequencing of T cell receptors in cutaneous T cell lymphoma. *Sci Transl Med,* 2013. 5(214): p. 214ra171.

[47] Wood, B., et al., Measurable residual disease detection by high-throughput sequencing improves risk stratification for pediatric B-ALL. *Blood,* 2018. 131(12): p. 1350-1359.

[48] Martinez-Lopez, J., et al., Prognostic value of deep sequencing method for minimal residual disease detection in multiple myeloma. *Blood,* 2014. 123(20): p. 3073-9.

[49] Gibbs, J. D., et al., Utility of flow cytometry and gene rearrangement analysis in tissue and blood of patients with suspected cutaneous T-cell lymphoma. *Oncol Rep,* 2021. 45(1): p. 349-358.

[50] de Masson, A., et al., High-throughput sequencing of the T cell receptor beta gene identifies aggressive early-stage mycosis fungoides. *Sci Transl Med,* 2018. 10(440): p. 10 5894.

[51] Segundo-Val, I. S. and C. S. Sanz-Lozano, Introduction to the Gene Expression Analysis. *Methods Mol Biol,* 2016. 1434: p. 29-43.

[52] Tsang, H. F., et al., NanoString, a novel digital color-coded barcode technology: current and future applications in molecular diagnostics. *Expert Rev Mol Diagn,* 2017. 17(1): p. 95-103.

[53] Litvinov, I. V., et al., Gene expression analysis in Cutaneous T-Cell Lymphomas (CTCL) highlights disease heterogeneity and potential diagnostic and prognostic indicators. *Oncoimmunology,* 2017. 6(5): p. e1306618.

[54] Litvinov, I. V., et al., The Use of Transcriptional Profiling to Improve Personalized Diagnosis and Management of Cutaneous T-cell Lymphoma (CTCL). *Clin Cancer Res,* 2015. 21(12): p. 2820-9.

[55] Nebozhyn, M., et al., Quantitative PCR on 5 genes reliably identifies CTCL patients with 5% to 99% circulating tumor cells with 90% accuracy. *Blood,* 2006. 107(8): p. 3189-96.

[56] Michel, L., et al., Use of PLS3, Twist, CD158k/KIR3DL2, and NKp46 gene expression combination for reliable Sézary syndrome diagnosis. *Blood,* 2013. 121(8): p. 1477-8.

[57] Zhang, Y., et al., Molecular markers of early-stage mycosis fungoides. *J Invest Dermatol,* 2012. 132(6): p. 1698-706.

[58] Huang, Y., et al., Thymocyte selection-associated high mobility group box gene (TOX) is aberrantly over-expressed in mycosis fungoides

and correlates with poor prognosis. *Oncotarget,* 2014. 5(12): p. 4418-25.

[59] Bagot, M., New Targeted Treatments for Cutaneous T-cell Lymphomas. *Indian J Dermatol,* 2017. 62(2): p. 142-145.

[60] Van Der Weyden, C., et al., IPH4102, a monoclonal antibody directed against the immune receptor molecule KIR3DL2, for the treatment of cutaneous T-cell lymphoma. *Expert Opin Investig Drugs,* 2018. 27(8): p. 691-697.

[61] Kim, Y. H., et al., Mogamulizumab versus vorinostat in previously treated cutaneous T-cell lymphoma (MAVORIC): an international, open-label, randomised, controlled phase 3 trial. *Lancet Oncol,* 2018. 19(9): p. 1192-1204.

[62] O'Brien, J., et al., Overview of MicroRNA Biogenesis, Mechanisms of Actions, and Circulation. *Front Endocrinol* (Lausanne), 2018. 9: p. 402.

[63] Ralfkiaer, U., et al., MicroRNA expression in early mycosis fungoides is distinctly different from atopic dermatitis and advanced cutaneous T-cell lymphoma. *Anticancer Res,* 2014. 34(12): p. 7207-17.

[64] Ralfkiaer, U., et al., Diagnostic microRNA profiling in cutaneous T-cell lymphoma (CTCL). *Blood,* 2011. 118(22): p. 5891-900.

[65] Dusilkova, N., et al., Plasma miR-155, miR-203, and miR-205 are Biomarkers for Monitoring of Primary Cutaneous T-Cell Lymphomas. *Int J Mol Sci,* 2017. 18(10).

[66] Lindahl, L. M., et al., Prognostic miRNA classifier in early-stage mycosis fungoides: development and validation in a Danish nationwide study. *Blood,* 2018. 131(7): p. 759-770.

[67] Baslan, T. and J. Hicks, Unravelling biology and shifting paradigms in cancer with single-cell sequencing. *Nat Rev Cancer,* 2017. 17(9): p. 557-569.

[68] Lawson, D. A., et al., Tumour heterogeneity and metastasis at single-cell resolution. *Nat Cell Biol,* 2018. 20(12): p. 1349-1360.

[69] Gaydosik, A. M., et al., Single-Cell Lymphocyte Heterogeneity in Advanced Cutaneous T-cell Lymphoma Skin Tumors. *Clin Cancer Res,* 2019. 25(14): p. 4443-4454.

[70] Buus, T. B., et al., Single-cell heterogeneity in Sézary syndrome. *Blood Adv,* 2018. 2(16): p. 2115-2126.

[71] Borcherding, N., et al., Single-Cell Profiling of Cutaneous T-Cell Lymphoma Reveals Underlying Heterogeneity Associated with Disease Progression. *Clin Cancer Res,* 2019. 25(10): p. 2996-3005.

[72] da Silva Almeida, A. C., et al., The mutational landscape of cutaneous T cell lymphoma and Sézary syndrome. *Nat Genet,* 2015. 47(12): p. 1465-70.

[73] McGirt, L. Y., et al., Whole-genome sequencing reveals oncogenic mutations in mycosis fungoides. *Blood,* 2015. 126(4): p. 508-19.

[74] Choi, J., et al., Genomic landscape of cutaneous T cell lymphoma. *Nat Genet,* 2015. 47(9): p. 1011-9.

[75] Ungewickell, A., et al., Genomic analysis of mycosis fungoides and Sézary syndrome identifies recurrent alterations in TNFR2. *Nat Genet,* 2015. 47(9): p. 1056-60.

[76] Damsky, W. E. and J. Choi, Genetics of Cutaneous T Cell Lymphoma: From Bench to Bedside. *Curr Treat Options Oncol,* 2016. 17(7): p. 33.

[77] Wang, L., et al., Genomic profiling of Sézary syndrome identifies alterations of key T cell signaling and differentiation genes. *Nat Genet,* 2015. 47(12): p. 1426-34.

[78] Boonk, S. E., et al., Evaluation of Immunophenotypic and Molecular Biomarkers for Sézary Syndrome Using Standard Operating Procedures: A Multicenter Study of 59 Patients. *J Invest Dermatol,* 2016. 136(7): p. 1364-1372.

[79] Park, J., et al., Genomic analysis of 220 CTCLs identifies a novel recurrent gain-of-function alteration in RLTPR (p.Q575E). *Blood,* 2017. 130(12): p. 1430-1440.

[80] Perez, C., et al., Mutated JAK kinases and deregulated STAT activity are potential therapeutic targets in cutaneous T-cell lymphoma. *Haematologica,* 2015. 100(11): p. e450-3.

[81] Drosten, M. and M. Barbacid, Targeting the MAPK Pathway in KRAS-Driven Tumors. *Cancer Cell,* 2020. 37(4): p. 543-550.

[82] Halle, B. R. and D. B. Johnson, Defining and Targeting BRAF Mutations in Solid Tumors. *Curr Treat Options Oncol,* 2021. 22(4): p. 30.

[83] Lee, S., J. Rauch, and W. Kolch, Targeting MAPK Signaling in Cancer: Mechanisms of Drug Resistance and Sensitivity. *Int J Mol Sci,* 2020. 21(3).

[84] Sekulic, A., et al., Personalized treatment of Sézary syndrome by targeting a novel CTLA4:CD28 fusion. *Mol Genet Genomic Med,* 2015. 3(2): p. 130-6.

[85] Vaqué, J. P., et al., PLCG1 mutations in cutaneous T-cell lymphomas. *Blood,* 2014. 123(13): p. 2034-43.

[86] Chang, T. P., V. Poltoratsky, and I. Vancurova, Bortezomib inhibits expression of TGF-beta1, IL-10, and CXCR4, resulting in decreased survival and migration of cutaneous T cell lymphoma cells. *J Immunol,* 2015. 194(6): p. 2942-53.

[87] Sors, A., et al., Down-regulating constitutive activation of the NF-kappaB canonical pathway overcomes the resistance of cutaneous T-cell lymphoma to apoptosis. *Blood,* 2006. 107(6): p. 2354-63.

[88] Nicolay, J. P., et al., Dimethyl fumarate restores apoptosis sensitivity and inhibits tumor growth and metastasis in CTCL by targeting NF-kappaB. *Blood,* 2016. 128(6): p. 805-15.

[89] Zinzani, P. L., et al., Phase II trial of proteasome inhibitor bortezomib in patients with relapsed or refractory cutaneous T-cell lymphoma. *J Clin Oncol,* 2007. 25(27): p. 4293-7.

[90] van Doorn, R., et al., Epigenomic Analysis of Sézary Syndrome Defines Patterns of Aberrant DNA Methylation and Identifies Diagnostic Markers. *J Invest Dermatol,* 2016. 136(9): p. 1876-1884.

[91] Kiel, M. J., et al., Genomic analyses reveal recurrent mutations in epigenetic modifiers and the JAK-STAT pathway in Sézary syndrome. *Nat Commun,* 2015. 6: p. 8470.

[92] Stephens, P. J., et al., Massive genomic rearrangement acquired in a single catastrophic event during cancer development. *Cell,* 2011. 144(1): p. 27-40.

[93] Singhi, A. D., et al., Preoperative next-generation sequencing of pancreatic cyst fluid is highly accurate in cyst classification and detection of advanced neoplasia. *Gut,* 2018. 67(12): p. 2131-2141.
[94] Nikiforov, Y. E. and Z. W. Baloch, Clinical validation of the ThyroSeq v3 genomic classifier in thyroid nodules with indeterminate FNA cytology. *Cancer Cytopathol,* 2019. 127(4): p. 225-230.

In: Mycosis Fungoides and Sézary Syndrome ISBN: 978-1-68507-093-9
Editors: X. Zhang and L. Sokol

Chapter 9

TREATMENT OF MYCOSIS FUNGOIDES

Brandon Cardon, MD, David Aung-Din, MD and Lucia Seminario-Vidal*, MD, PhD

[1]Department of Dermatology and Cutaneous Surgery,
University of South Florida Morsani College of Medicine,
Tampa, FL, USA
[2]Department of Cutaneous Oncology,
H. Lee Moffitt Cancer Center and Research Institute,
Tampa, FL, USA

INTRODUCTION

Mycosis fungoides (MF) is characterized with a chronic, relapsing course that can require multiple and consecutive therapies [1]. Consideration needs to be made in regards to symptom severity, other co-existing symptoms (i.e., pruritus) and patient-specific circumstances (age, co-morbidities) [1]. Subtype of MF also becomes important to treatment choice, as folliculotropic MF (FMF) can generally be less responsive to certain skin-

* Corresponding Author's Email: luciasem@usf.edu.

directed therapies [2]. Treatment goals include clearance of skin disease, limiting recurrence, prevention of progression and quality of life [1]. In patients with limited patch-plaque stage MF, one or more topical formulations can provide excellent response rate and prognosis [1]. Many options for skin-directed therapies (SDT) are available, which include topical corticosteroids, mechlormethamine, retinoids, phototherapy and radiotherapy [3]. With widespread patch-plaque disease, phototherapy is often required [1]. Refractory MF and FMF can often require a combination of SDT and other systemic therapies [1, 3]. Systemic therapies have recently evolved, and now include monoclonal antibodies, such as brentuximab and mogamulizumab, as well as older treatment options, such as systemic retinoids, histone deacetylase inhibitors, and interferon [3]. A new understanding of the pathogenesis of MF and discovery of important molecular markers has led to the increased development of targeted therapies that are being investigated in clinical trials for MF [1].

SKIN-DIRECTED THERAPIES

Topical Corticosteroids

Topical corticosteroids (TCS) (Table 9-1) have first been reported in the treatment of MF since the 1960s [3]. They are the most common treatment used in early MF and can be used as adjunctive treatment to all other therapies [1]. TCS have multiple targeted effects, including the induction of apoptosis, affecting T-lymphocyte adhesion to endothelium and transcript factor downregulation [1]. Large prospective studies of patients with patch stage disease treated with almost always twice daily topical class I through class III steroids revealed complete responses in 63% of T1 and 25% of T2 patients with median observation time of 9 months [4]. However, cutaneous side effects of TCS are common [3]. Recent studies have reported that 10-20% of patients using class I TCS for greater than three months developed an irritant dermatitis or purpura [3]. Long term side effects can also include skin atrophy, hypopigmentation, striae and potential systemic absorption

[1]. Systemic absorption was observed in one study without any adrenal suppression [1]. Sustained responses to topical steroids were not observed after discontinuation of therapy [1, 5]. Current recommendation is to use higher potency class TCS over lower potency, as these are mostly well-tolerated with minimal risk of adverse effects if used with other inflammatory regimens [3].

Table 9-1. Examples of common topical corticosteroids

Potency	Name	Formulation
Superpotent	Betamethasone dipropionate	0.05% ointment
	Clobetasol	0.05% cream or ointment
	Diforasone diacetate	0.05% ointment
	Halobetasol propionate	0.05% cream or ointment
High potency	Amcinonide	0.1% ointment
	Betamethasone dipropionate	0.05% cream
	Desoximetasone	0.25% cream or ointment
	Fluocinonide	0.05% cream or ointment
	Halcinonide	0.1% cream
	Mometasone furoate	0.1% ointment
	Betamethasone valerate	0.1% ointment
	Diflorasone diacetate	0.05% cream
	Fluticasone propionate	0.005% ointment
	Triamcinolone	0.1% ointment
Mid potency	Fluocinolone acetonide	0.025% ointment
	Flurandrenonide	0.05% ointment
	Hydrocortisone valerate	0.2% ointment
	Triamcinolone	0.1% cream
	Hydrocortisone butyrate	0.1% cream
Low potency	Alcometasone dipropionate	0.05% cream or ointment
	Desonide	0.05% cream or ointment
	Flucinolone acetonide	0.01% cream
	Hydrocortisone acetate	0.5% cream or ointment

Topical Imidazoquinolines

Topical imiquimod is a toll-like-receptor-7 (TLR-7) agonist with both properties against viruses and tumors [3]. Use of these medications leads to production of interferon-α, tumor-necrosis-factor-α, interleukin-1 and interleukin-6 which can induce tumor cell apoptosis and death [3]. Recent studies of limited patient case series (20 patients) have demonstrated an overall response rate of 80%, with 45% of patients achieving complete response with imiquimod 5% [6]. Side effects are usually limited to the skin, including local irritation, pain, redness, pruritus, and even ulceration [3]. Rare reports exist of patients experiencing fatigue and flu-like symptoms with topical imiquimod [3]. However, most adverse effects resolve after a few weeks of treatment or with short treatment vacations [3].

Resiquimod is a similar agent, acting as a potent agonist of toll-like-receptor-7 and -8, which leads to production of interferon-α, interleukin-12 and interleukin-15 [7]. In limited phase I trials with 12 patients with stage IA-IIA MF, treatment with formulations of 0.03% and 0.06% resiquimod gel at dosing of once per day three times weekly (adjusted to 1, 2, 3, 5 or 7 times weekly based on tolerability) resulted in improvement of 75% of treated lesions [7]. Notably, three patients experienced responses in untreated lesions as well, which may suggest some systemic response [3]. As with imiquimod, adverse effects were mostly limited to the skin; however, two patients developed systemic effects in the form of fever [3]. Studies of the cell populations revealed that 90% of patients demonstrated a decrease of malignant T-cells in treated lesions [3].

Topical Mechlorethamine

Mechlorethamine hydrochloride is a nitrogen mustard that is one of the most studied treatments for MF [3]. Mechorethamine is an alkylating agent that induces DNA damage, which results in systemic anti-tumor effects, however, when used topically, may affect immune mechanisms involving keratinocyte, Langerhans cell, and T-cell interactions [1, 3]. Topical mechlorethamine is a first-line therapy for both local and generalized MF [3]. The efficacy of mechlorethamine in both aqueous solutions or ointments has been well-reported, at concentrations of either 0.01% or 0.02% [1]. Complete response has been demonstrated in up to 72% of patients with early-stage MF with occasional long-term remission periods of longer than 8 years [1]. Median time to complete response has been described to encompass 6–12-month periods [3]. A recent large multicenter trial had similar results, which led to the approval of mechlormethamine 0.02% gel by the FDA for the treament of stage IA/IB MF patients on previous SDT [1]. Used once daily, the overall response rate was 58.5%, with 13.8% of patients achieving complete response; 85.5% of patients had ongoing responses at 12 months; however, only 11% of these patients experienced CR after 10 years [1, 8]. While skin clearance is usually followed with maintenance therapy, there currently exists no evidence that prolonged maintenance therapy affects recurrence rates [1]. As with the previously described therapies, side effects are usually minor and limited to the skin [3]. Cutaneous side effects commonly reported include burning, pruritus, and irritant or allergic contact dermatitis [1, 3]. Incidents of allergic contact dermatitis are more commonly reported in aqueous formulations [1]. Decreasing frequency or concentrations of mechlorethamine, as well as concurrent use of TCS may improve tolerance [1, 3]. A small increased risk of developing non-melanoma skin cancers, especially with concurrent radiation or ultraviolet A phototherapy has also been described, as there are reports of MF patients without significant risk factors developing skin cancer [1, 3]. However, one study has demonstrated no significant increase in secondary skin cancers with long-term mechlorethamine treatment [3].

Topical Retinoids (Bexarotene, Tazarotene)

Topical bexarotene is a synthetic retinoid approved by the FDA for the treatment of early-stage MF [1]. Oral bexarotene functions primarily by selectively binding retinoid X receptors, affecting cellular differentiation and induction of apoptosis. However, topical bexarotene has a less clear mechanism [1]. It has been reported to induce apoptosis in MF cell lines [3]. Topical bexarotene 1% gel is recommended to be applied twice daily, but is FDA-approved for up to 4 times daily administration [1]. High rates of local irritation can be seen with 4 times daily regimen [1]. Phase I/II trials of topical bexarotene gel involved 67 patients with stage IA/IIA MF and demonstrated an overall response rate of 63% with complete response in 21% of patients [9]. 87% of patients reported local cutaneous adverse effects, including rash, pruritus, pain and eruption of a vesiculobullous rash [9].

Tazarotene is another topical retinoid that binds retinoic acid receptors-b and -y, which causes anti-proliferative and anti-inflammatory effects locally in the skin [1, 4]. In a study ten patients with early-stage MF were treated with tazarotene 0.1% cream to index lesions every other day for 2 weeks, then once daily for 6 months [10]. 60% of the patients experienced complete response, with mean time to complete response of 3.8 months [10]. However, 70% of patients reported grade I or grade II side effects, including erythema, burning, pruritus and desquamation [10]. Two patients withdrew from the study due to adverse effects [10]. Topical tazarotene 0.1% gel has also been studied as an adjuvant therapy in a population of 19 patients [11]. Overall response rate of 58% was observed in once daily applications for 24 weeks; however, local skin irritation was reported in 84% of the patients [11].

Topical Carmustine

Carmustine is an alkylating agent that causes DNA cross-linking, resulting in apoptosis [3]. Carmustine can be both compounded in aqueous or ointment formulations [5]. Studies of MF treated with topical carmustine at dosing variable from 2 mg/mL up to 60 mg daily revealed an overall response rate of 98% in patients with T1 and CR rate of 86% [12]. In patients with stage IB disease, overall response rate was 84% with CR rate of 47%. Median time to CR was 11.5 weeks [12]. Compared with mechlorethamine, carmustine causes less hypersensitivity reactions reported in only 5% to 10%

of cases [5]. Telangiectasias have been reported to develop in areas of prior erythema, which can be permanent [4]. The main risk of topical carmustine is systemic absorption, reported in up to 28% of patients, which can predispose patients to myelosuppression [5]. Due to this risk, monthly monitoring of complete blood counts is recommended [5, 12].

Topical Calcineurin Inhibitors

Topical calcineurin inhibitors (tacrolimus, pimecrolimus) are a class of immodulators that have begun to be investigated in management of MF [13]. Tacrolimus and other topical calcineurin inhibitors (TCI) work through inhibition of T-cells and the release of inflammatory cytokines and mediators [13, 14]. Investigations into PLCG1 and the nuclear factor of activated T-cells (NFAT) demonstrated that TCI resulted in antiproliferative and apoptotic responses [15]. A case report of a single patient with patch-stage MF showed CR with the use of topical tacrolimus ointment 0.1% twice daily for one month. Three months after response, the patient experienced relapse, which was successfully treated with the same regimen [13]. Another pediatric case with hypopigmented MF was successfully treated with a combination of topical corticosteroids 3 times weekly, narrow-band ultraviolet B phototherapy 2-3 times weekly and tacrolimus 2 times weekly [16]. Currently, a phase II clinical trial in Spain is being undertaken to evaluate the response of early-stage MF with topical pimecrolimus in 40 patients. After 16 weeks of treatment, response rate of 54% was reported, with one patient demonstrating CR [17]. Major adverse events reported with TCI include burning and pruritus [18]. There is a yet unclear and controversial risk of theoretical association with malignancies, including lymphoma, which existed as a boxed warning on these medications, which is not currently supported by the American Academy of Dermatology and other organizations [14].

Dosing

After choosing a topical medication, prescribing the correct amount to sufficiently cover the approximate body surface area involved is paramount to ensuring medication adherence and avoiding overuse. By using the Finger Tip Unit model first published by *Long* et al. prescribers can provide the sufficient amount of medication to treat affected areas as described below (Table 9-2) [19]:

Table 9-2. Calculating topical dose needed for treatment (in adults)

Body part	Finger Tip Unit (FTU)A	Gram equivalent for once daily dosing	Grams equivalent for twice daily dosing
Face and neck	2.5	1.25	2.5
Front of trunk	7	3.5	7
Back of trunk	7	3.5	7
Arm and forearm	3	1.5	3
Hand	1	0.5	1
Leg and thigh	6	3	6
Foot	2	1	2

A. Each FTU is the equivalent of 0.5 g and is the amount of ointment applied from the distal skin crease to the tip of the index finger.

Local and Generalized Radiation

Mycosis fungoides is a highly radiosensitive disease, and therapy with radiation can be effective in most stages of MF [3]. When the disease is limited to patch/plaque stage, topicals or phototherapy are first-line therapies; however, when tumors are present, local control can be achieved with radiation therapy [20]. For local palliation, ultra-low doses

(2Gy times 2 series) can achieve a complete response rate, but higher doses (>8 Gy) achieve >90% complete response rates [20]. Tumor stage disease or large-cell transformation can require higher doses [20]. In patients who have difficulties with accessing therapy, treatment can be performed in a single fraction, with a significant complete response rate of 94.4% [3]. Side effects of local radiation are dependent on dosing, and at very low doses (2Gy), radiation therapy has essentially no side effects [3]. At higher doses, side effects are minimal; most commonly reported side effects include dryness, atrophy, erythema and desquamation at target sites [3]. Local radiotherapy may also have a role in stage III to IVA erythrodermic MF if isolated tumors are present or there is severe involvement of the distal extremities [5].

Total skin electron beam therapy (TSEBT) can be used in MF patients with extensive patches and plaques at any stage [5]. TSEBT involves the use of ionizing radiation to the entire surface of the skin, that results in deeper penetration compared to nitrogen mustards or phototherapy [1]. TSEBT is a technically challenging approach of radiation that requires a large electron field or a rotational technique to ensure total skin coverage and protective measures such as shielding of eyes and nailbeds [20]. Conventional TSEBT involves 30-36 Gy ionizing radiation over a period of eight to ten weeks, leading to complete response in 75% of T2 and 47% T3 MF [21]. The median duration of these responses was 29 months for T2 and 9 months for T3 disease [21]. Repeat courses are limited due to potential skin toxicity and necrosis [1]. Subsequent SDT or systemic agents have shown mixed results [1]. A second TSEBT course at lower dose can be considered in select populations based on initial dose, tolerance, and length of time between doses [21]. TSEBT toxicity is generally dose-dependent and can include xerosis, erythema and desquamation, with long term effects on nails (dystrophy, nail loss), alopecia, anhidrosis and skin atrophy/necrosis [1]. Low dose radiation of 10 Gy may decrease side effects and enable repeat radiation; however lower response rates and durations are seen with reduced doses [1].

Local and Generalized Phototherapy (UVB, NBUVB, Excimer, PUVA/UVA1, PDT)

Phototherapy has been a mainstay of therapy for MF for several decades [17]. Specifically, ultraviolet B (UVB) and psoralen plus ultraviolet A (PUVA) have initially been used as monotherapy for early-stage MF but have more recently been expanded with combination of systemic treatments [22]. The United States Cutaneous Lymphoma Consortium recommends phototherapy for patients with early-stage MF and in combination with systemic therapy in patients with refractory or advanced disease [3]. Historically, broadband UVB therapy was widely used, but now most phototherapy is used in the form of narrow band (NB) UVB [21]. Other types of phototherapy, including excimer, UVA1, and photodynamic therapy have also been supported in reports as treatment for MF [3]. Phototherapy treatment protocols include clearance, consolidation, and maintenance phases [3]. After 100% clearance has been achieved, patients may benefit from a consolidation phase lasting approximately one to three months prior to initiating lower maintenance regimens [3]. It is theorized that the consolidation phase may increase histological and molecular clearance and loss of the dominant T-cell, which may not correlate with skin clearance [3]. A prolonged maintenance phase after clearance may have some benefit in prolonging relapse time and decreasing relapse-rates, but it remains controversial due to the lack of significant data from randomized prospective studies as well as the risk of increased UV exposure [3].

Contraindications to phototherapy include any co-existing photosensitive disorder (xeroderma pigmentosa, lupus, and porphyrias) [3]. PUVA should not be used in patients with a history of melanoma or multiple non-melanoma skin cancers or in pregnant or lactating women. Chronic actinic dermatitis and claustrophobia are relative contraindications to phototherapy [3]. Caution is advised in children, immunosuppressed patients, or patients on photosensitizing medications, such as tetracyclines or NSAIDs [3]. Common side effects of active phototherapy include erythema and pruritus, especially during PUVA [3]. Photo damage has also been reported as a side effect, also particularly with PUVA, with at least

27% of MF patients showing signs of photodamage [3]. Development of secondary skin cancers is another potentially serious side effect of phototherapy [3]. In general, the risk of skin cancer is not significantly increased with UVB therapy; however it is reported that there may be an increase in basal cell carcinomas and skin cancers of the genitals in patients on both UVB and PUVA [3]. Patients who receive PUVA do have an increased risk of skin cancer, in particular squamous cell carcinoma and basal cell carcinoma [3]. A long-term cohort study of 66 MF patients that received PUVA revealed that 26% of the patients had developed skin cancer that was diagnosed as Bowen disease, squamous or basal cell carcinoma. One patient developed melanoma in situ, and another developed metastatic melanoma during maintenance treatment [22].

UVB phototherapy units emit light with a wavelength between 270 to 390 nm with a peak of 313 nm [21]. NB-UVB has a sharp emission peak between 311 nm and 312 nm [22]. Due to the shorter wavelength, UVB has less depth of penetration as compared to UVA. UVB suppresses neoplastic T-cell functions and proliferation by inhibiting antigen-presenting cells and increases local cytokine production from keratinocytes [1]. NBUVB is used more frequently than PUVA in early-stage MF because of its similar efficacies and its decreased rate of skin cancer as compared to PUVA [1]. Most centers recommend treatment sessions of two to three times weekly for practical convenience [22]. Starting dose is determined from the minimal erythema dose or by skin type [22]. The minimal erythema dose is normally utilized in a reported history of sensitivity to the sun [22]. Published reports of complete response for NB-UVB range from 54%-90% in patients with stage IA-IIA disease [22]. Patients with patch disease responded better than those with plaque stage [22].

PUVA utilizes oral 8-methoxypsoralen, which sensitizes the skin to UVA radiation at 320-400 nm, causing induction of tumor cell apoptosis, DNA damage, suppression cytokine production, and depletion of Langerhans cells [1]. PUVA may be more beneficial in patients with thicker plaques, FMF, or darker skin tones [3]. Topical methoxalen (1%) is also available for localized treatment [21]. Like UVB, PUVA treatments are given two to three times weekly and starting doses are based on skin type

[22]. MF patients can also undergo maintenance treatments as in NBUVB, but this is controversial [5]. It remains uncertain if maintenance PUVA prolongs remission [5]. A solitary retrospective analysis of early-stage MF patients having achieved remission with PUVA monotherapy concluded that 30-50% of patients had prolonged remission of ~10-year disease-free survival rates, but most of these patients received maintenance therapy [5, 23]. Complete response rates of PUVA have been reported as 85% for stage IA, 65% for stage IB, and 85% for stage IIA patients [5]. With the reports of increased risk of skin cancers, the British Association of Dermatologists recommends limiting cumulative exposure to 1,200 J/cm^2 or 250 total sessions and recommends avoiding maintenance PUVA [5].

UVA1 is longwave phototherapy which penetrates the skin at the level of the dermis and does not require psoralen as adjunct therapy [3]. This in turn results in lower phototoxicity as compared to PUVA [3]. There have been small studies of use of UVA1 for early-stage MF; the largest with 19 patients receiving 30 J/cm2 five times weekly for five weeks [3]. Sixty-three percent (63%) of patients experienced CR and 37% experienced partial response [5]. Relapses were reported to have occurred in 58% of patients within three months of finishing therapy [3]. With limited toxicity, UVA1 may be a safer alternative to other SDT [3].

There are several reports that support the use of monochromatic excimer light of 308 nm for patch stage MF [3]. Two series demonstrated high response rates with one study reported four of four total patients with complete response, both histologic and clinical response [3]. However, in both series, follow-up times were short [3]. Excimer may serve a useful role for sites that are not easily accessible, such as acral or intertriginous areas [3].

Photodynamic therapy uses visible light to activate a photosensitizing agent, resulting in the creation of reactive oxygen species and cause cell death in affected cells [3]. Photodynamic therapy has demonstrated efficacy in the treatment of actinic keratoses and non-melanoma skin cancer [3]. The most common photosensitizing agent is 5-aminolevulinic acid [3]. A small case series of 10 patients with plaque and tumor lesions underwent this therapy [3]. Seven (7) out of 9 treated plaques had a complete clinical response; however, tumors demonstrated no response [3]. A common side effect of PDT is local pain. One of the patients in the above series dropped out due to pain, and most patients reported local edema and erythema [3].

Systemic Therapies

Although MF is limited to skin involvement, systemic therapy is appropriate in many circumstances (Table 9-3 and Table 9-4). The NCCN guidelines recommend several stages of MF be considered for systemic therapy. This includes patients with limited skin involvement T1A (<10% BSA) who experience inadequate response to multiple previous skin-directed therapies, stage IB/IIA (>10%BSA) with higher skin disease burden, or large plaque involvement or stage IIB with even limited tumor burden. Increased severity stage IIB disease with heavy tumor burden as well as stage III and IV disease can always be considered for systemic therapy [24].

There are many novel agents and targets for MF/Sézary syndrome (SS) (Fig. 9-1). Chimeric Antigen Receptor (CAR) T-cell therapy has had many hurdles in becoming a viable treatment for CTCL including T-cell aplasia, fratricide, and product contamination. Targets have included CD4 and CD30 expressed in T-cell lymphomas as well as CCR4 (similarly targeted by mogalizumab), a chemokine receptor expressed abundantly in CTCL [23]. TTI-621 (SIRPαFc) is a novel CD47 decoy receptor that links to CD47, abundantly overexpressed in Sézary cells. CD47 typically leads to protection against macrophage phagocytosis providing "do-not-eat-me" signal. SIRPαFc blocks this receptor and provides a linkage point for macrophages to recognize and phagocytize the tumor cells [25]. IPH402-101 is an anti-KIR3DL2 (CD158k) monoclonal antibody expressed in CTCL and specifically SS [26]. MRG 106 is a locked nucleic acid-modified oligonucleotide inhibitor of miR-155, a micro-RNA found to be associated with poor prognosis in CTCL. Inhibition of this miRNA is reported to reduce several downstream survival pathways including JAK/STAT, MAPK/ERK, and PI3K/AKT [27]. Pembrolizumab is an anti-PD1 monoclonal antibody (programmed cell death receptor) and immune checkpoint inhibitor being studied as an option for patients with MF/SS, especially those with refractory disease [28]. Immunotoxins are another class of medications; these therapies contain two components: a target-specific binding domain that binds to a cell surface marker and a cytotoxic domain that binds to the cell surface marker and enters the cell leading to apoptosis. Therapies in this class include a pseudomonas exotoxin linked to a CD25 antibody (LMB-2), diphtheria toxin fused with IL-2 (denileukin difitox), and a diptheria toxin linked to a CD3ε antibody (anti-CD3 immunotoxin, A-dmDT390-bisFv(UCHT1)) [29]. BNZ-1 is a pegylated peptide antagonist that binds to the common γc signaling receptor for the cytokines IL-2, IL-9, and IL-15. Inhibition of these interleukins is proposed to downregulate survival pathways in CTCL tumor cells including the JAK/STAT pathway leading to an anti-tumor response [30]. Duvelisib (IPI-145) is an oral inhibitor of phosphatidylinositol 3-kinase (PI3K)–δ/γ isoforms, a lipid kinase molecule which is proposed to have several downstream signaling effects that lead to anti-tumor properties [31].

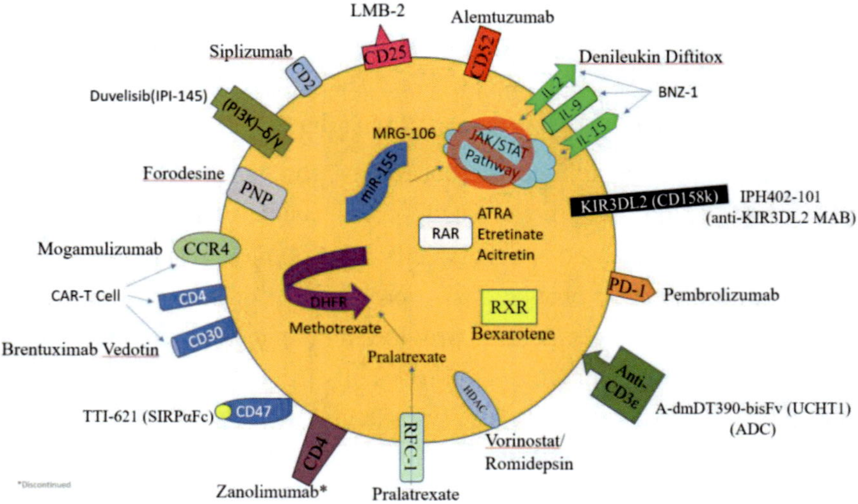

Figure 9-1. Systemic therapies and their targets.

Table 9-3. Preferred regimens

Agent	Mechanism	Most Common Adverse Effects	Examples of Treatment Regimen
Systemic Retinoids (Acitretin, Etretinate, Isotretinoin, Bexarotene)	Bind Nuclear Receptors Retinoic Acid Receptors (RAR) and Retinoid X Receptor (RXR)	Mucocutaneous, GI Disturbances, Hair Loss, myalgia, arthralgia, headache including pseudotumor cerebri, hypertriglyceridemia, Elevated LFT's, Hypothyroidism, Teratogenicity, Leukopenia, agranulocytosis	Acitretin- RAR 32 patients, most received 25 mg daily, overall response rate 59% (19 patients), 1 with CR and 18 with PR, median duration of response 28 months [32]. Etretinate-RAR, Isotretinoin-RAR- Reviews show overall response rates from 43% to 100%, complete response 12-30% over 3-15 months [33]. ATRA-All-Trans Retinoic Acid)-RAR, Alternate days of IV infusions reports of unpublished data inducing remission in 2 patients [34]. Bexarotene-All RXR 300 mg/m2/day led to overall response rate of 48%, 4% CR and 23% had a 75-100% response [35].
Methotrexate	Binds dihydrofolate (DHFR) reductase which prevents conversion of DHF to tetrahydrofolate, results in decreased purine synthesis, and decreased cell division	Oral mucositis, GI, myelodepression, neurologic, LFT elevation, pneumonitis, skin eruptions	Erythrodermic CTCL Dose from 5-125 mg Qweekly, 41% CR 17% PR ORR 58%, median freedom from treatment failure 31 months [36]. T2 Disease Median dose 25 mg, up to 50 mg weekly 12% CR 22% PR, ORR 33%,time to treatment failure 15 months [37].

Table 9-3. (Continued)

Agent	Mechanism	Most Common Adverse Effects	Examples of Treatment Regimen
Interferons	Naturally occurring polypeptides part of Innate Immune system, that work through several immunomodulatory pathways IFN-Alpha and IFN-Gamma are most commonly used	Fever, fatigue, weight loss, neutropenia, elevated LDH, elevated LFT's, skin eruptions, nephrotic syndrome	IFN-Gamma PR in 31% lasted median of 10 months, 0% CR, median dose of 0.5 mg/m2 per day [38]. IFN-Alpha CR in 27% (mean time 21 weeks), PR in 45% (mean 8 weeks), patients either received 3 million IU or were escalated to 36 million IU IM daily for 10 week induction [39].
Extracorporeal Photopheresis (ECP)	Pheresis performed, blood separated into leukocytes and RBC's. 8-methoxypsoralen is added to leukocytes and radiated with UVA, which is then infused back into patient, leading to immunomodulatory effects on T-Cells, exact MOA is not clearly understood	Headache, fever, shivering, nausea, photosensitivity, hypotension, CHF, tachycardia	17 patients with stage 1-2 and 33 patients with stage 3-4, average of 39 cycles with overall response rate of 42%, overall survival of 72 months, median time to response 11 months [40]. Generalized Erythroderma or extensive patch-plaque Patients with ORR 74%, 33% PR, 41% ≥90% improvement after median of 19.6 months, mean of 40 ECP treatments, Median OS 9.2 years from diagnosis 6.6 years from ECP initiation [41].

Table 9-4. Other agents

Agent	Mechanism	Efficacy	Toxicity
Chlorambucil	Alkylating agent that cross-links DNA during all phases of the cell cycle	Commonly used outside the USA as first-line therapy for advanced stages, but large-scale clinical trial data as to its efficacy is lacking [58]. A study of 13 patients with erythrodermic CTCl treated with pulsed chlorambucil and corticosteroids demonstrated 7/13 CR and 6/13 PR [59].	In the pulsed chlorambucil/corticosteroid study, no therapy-related severe (grades 2–4) or treatment-limiting side-effects occurred [59].
Pembrolizumab	Target the programmed cell-death-1 (PD-1) receptor. PD-1 is expressed on follicular helper T-cells, and functions to promote self-tolerance by promoting apoptosis of antigen-specific T-cells while enhancing T-cell regulatory function	PD-1 expression is high in patch and plaque-stage MF [58]. In a phase II clinical trial of 24 patients with advanced-stage MF ORR was 38% with two complete responses and seven partial responses [28].	No reported grade 4 or 5 adverse events. Total of 11 adverse effects of any grade were observed among nine patients. Four patients discontinued treatment due to grade 3 adverse events including pneumonitis, duodenitis, transaminits, and corneal ulcer. An additional patient discontinued treatment after completion of the trial due to development of grade 2 colitis 24 months into treatment. [28].
Pentostatin	Inhibitor of adenosine deaminase; selectively toxic to lymphocytes [61].	ORR of 39% in 18 patients with stage I to IVB CTCL treated with 4 to 5 mg/m2 of intravenous pentostatin every 1 to 4 weeks. Two patients had CRs with a duration of response of 4 months to 6 years and 5 patients had PRs lasting for 1.5 to 6 months [61]. Also reported is a 40% OR rate and 7% CR rate in 94 CTCL patients treated with pentostatin studied in multicenter phase II trials. The median time to progression ranged from 1.3 to 8.3 months [62]	Toxicities include hematologic, renal insufficiency, nausea, and conjunctivitis. Also associated with angina and myocardial infarction, heart failure, and acute arrhythmias in patients with conditions such as coronary artery disease, congestive heart failure, hypertension, and pulmonary metastases [60].

Table 9-4. (Continued)

Agent	Mechanism	Efficacy	Toxicity
Temozolomide	Oral imidazotetrazine derivative of the alkylating agent dacarbazine [63]	Phase II study investigating the use of temozolomide (5-d dosing regimen of 200 mg/m2) in 29 patients with stage IIb–IVa MF. Reported moderate activity with an overall response rate of 27% and median disease-free survival of four months [63] Four patients reported using oral temozolomide (200 mg/m2 daily for 5/28 d) for CNS relapse of MF with one complete response, one partial response, and two demonstrations of stable disease. Oral temozolomide following whole-brain irradiation appears to have efficacy in patients with CNS progression of MF [64]	In the phase II trial, the most frequent adverse effects included constitutional symptoms, gastrointestinal symptoms, and hematologic toxicities. Three patients experienced grade 3 thrombocytopenia, lymphopenia, and skin reaction and treatment was discontinued [63]. Formal toxicity data were not accurately collected in all cases. However, none of the four patients required a dose reduction or stopped treatment as a result of toxicity [64].
Bortezomib	20S proteasome inhibitor	Phase II trial in 12 relapsed/refractory CTCL and 2 PTCLU reported an ORR of 67% and a CR rate of 17% [65].	No grade 4 toxicity reported. Grade 3 neutropenia was recorded in two patients, grade 3 thrombocytopenia was observed in 2 patients. The most significant toxicity was sensory neuropathy: grade 1 to 3 was observed in 50% of patients, but only one patient reported grade 3 toxicity with complete recovery within 6 weeks [65].

Agent	Mechanism	Efficacy	Toxicity
Gemcitabine	Nucleoside analog of pyridine nucleoside that inhibits DNA synthesis	Phase II study of 25 CTCL patients, with reported ORR of 68% and a CR rate of 8% [66].	Myelosuppression, hemolytic uremic syndrome, pulmonary embolism, and 1 episode each of congestive heart failure, acute myocardial infarction, and stable angina were observed. Increased hepatic transaminases, lethargy, fever, cutaneous hyperpigmentation, infusion-related maculopapular rash and radiation recall also reported [66].
Pralatrexate	Inhibits dihydrofolate reductase, resulting in disruption of DNA synthesis and tumor cell death [68]	In the Pralatrexate in Patients with Relapsed or Refractory Peripheral T-cell Lymphoma (PROPEL) prospective study, 12 patients studied with transformed MF. ORR was 25% by independent central review with a median DoR of 2.2 months [58]. A recent cohort study of 54 CTCL patients using a novel de-escalation praltrexate dosing schedule. Twenty-nine patients in the expansion cohort using the recommended dosage demonstrated 45% ORR [67].	Most common adverse events reported in the PROPEL study were mucositis (22–58%), fatigue (43%), nausea (39%), and thrombocytopenia (32%) [58]. In the cohort study, the only grade 4 adverse event was leukopenia (3%). The most common grade 3 adverse event was mucositis (17%) [67]
Doxorubicin	Anthracycline	ORR of 41–88%, and a time to relapse of 13 months [58].	Adverse effects include cardiotoxicity, cytopenia, GI symptoms, palmoplantar erythrodysesthesia, and alopecia [68]

THERAPIES FOR RELAPSED OR REFRACTORY DISEASE

Guidelines to evaluate disease response have been published for standardized assessment of MF [42]. Assessing response to treatment depends on the initial staging of MF and routine re-evaluation [42]. Progression in skin-limited disease is defined as >25% increase in skin disease from baseline, new tumors present in patients in T1, T2, or T4 (skin only) disease, or loss of response in those with partial or complete response [42]. Progression in disease with lymph node involvement is defined as a greater than 50% increase in the sum of the product of the longest bidimensional diameters (SPD), any new node that fits criteria and is proven to be N3 histologically, or a loss of response in patients with previous partial response [42]. Similarly, in organ involvement, there is >50% increase in SPD of any organs involved, new organ evolvement, or loss of response (>50% increase from the nadir in size of any previous organ involvement) [42]. In patients with blood involvement, any progression from B0 to B2, >50% increase from baseline and at least 5,000 neoplastic cells/μL, and loss of response in those with PR who were originally B2 at baseline, > 50% increase from nadir and at least 5,000 neoplastic cells/μL will meet criteria for progression [42]. Relapse is defined as any skin lesion recurrence, any new lymph node >1.5 cm histologically proven N3, new organ involvement, or increase of neoplastic blood lymphocytes to B1 or greater in a patient with previous CR [42].

Histone Deacetylase Inhibitors

Vorinostat is a histone deacetylase (HDAC) inhibitor that restores the expression of tumor suppressor or cell cycle regulatory genes by increasing histone acetylation. Vorinostate is approved by the FDA for CTCL that has progressed beyond stage IB and is refractory to 2 systemic therapies [1]. Vorinostat also inactivates STAT3 which is expressed in MF and can enhance the retinoid effects of RAR/RXR activation and transcription. Phase 2 trial of vorinostat demonstrated partial response in 29.7% of 74 patients.

All patients received 400 mg of vorinostat daily, which could be reduced to 300 mg daily for toxicity [43]. A similar phase 2 trial of 33 pretreated MF patients found that sustained 400 mg dosing was more efficacious and less toxic than 300 mg twice daily regimens, with a similar overall response rate of 24.2% [44]. The MAVORIC phase III trial evaluated response of MF/SS patients treated with vorinostat vs. mogamulizumab and revealed superior progression-free survival with mogamulizumab (median 7.7 months) compared with vorinostat therapy (median 3.1 months) [45].

Romidepsin inhibits class I and II HDACs and is intravenously administered at a weekly dose of 14 mg/m^2 for 3 weeks with 1 week off, and continued until intolerance or progression [1]. It received FDA approval for advanced CTCL that is refractory to ≥1 systemic therapy [1]. Two phase II trials have evaluated romidepsin in advanced-stage MF, with 1 showing a 38% response rate out of 68 patients including 5 patients with CR [46]. The other phase II trial observed complete responses in four patients, and partial responses were observed in 20 patients for an overall response rate of 34% in a total of 71 patients [47]. Pruritus reduction has been reported but may not correlate with objective clinical response [48]. Most reported side effects were gastrointestinal disturbances such as nausea or anorexia, hematologic abnormalities (anemia, thrombocytopenia, neutropenia, lymphopenia), and infectious complications [1]. EKG assessments also noted T wave flattening in 71% of patients, with less common ST depression and rare QTc prolongations [1].

Antibodies

Brentuximab vedotin (BV) is a CD30 specific antibody-drug conjugate specific for human CD30. With its high specificity for CD30, BV is an ideal treatment for CD30 expressing malignancies such as anaplastic large cell lymphoma [49].

Two phase-II clinical trials investigated the efficacy of BV in patients with CTCL. In the first study, 32 patients with MF and SS with variable CD30 expression were treated every three weeks for a maximum of 16 cycles with an overall response rate of 70% (21 of 30 patients; 2 patients did not have available efficacy evaluations) [50]. Patients with less than 5% CD30 expression had a lower rate of overall response than did those with 5% or more CD30 expression [50]. In the second study, the efficacy and safety of brentuximab was studied in 48 patients with CD30+ lymphoproliferative disorders or MF with the same dose and treatment schedule. The overall response rate was 73% with complete response of 35% reported, with a median response duration of 32 weeks. The overall response rate of the 28 MF patients was 54%, compared to the 100% response rate of CD30+ lymphoproliferative group. MF patients with different CD30 expression (low, moderate, and high) had a similar overall response rate of 50–58%; however complete responses were seen in the moderate and high groups, and the only patient with progressive disease had low expression of CD30 [51]. Peripheral neuropathy was the most common side effect. In the second study, grade 1 and grade 2 neuropathy developed in 31 of the 48 patients (67%) [51]. In randomized, multicenter phase III study (ALCANZA) of BV versus investigator choice (oral MTX or oral bexarotene), global response rate lasting at least 4 months was reported in 56.3% of patients treated with BV versus 12.5% treated with physician's choice. Higher grade (3-4) adverse events were observed in 41% of patients in BV arm and 47% in physician's choice arm. Peripheral neuropathy was reported in 67% of patients treated with BV vs. 4% in the control arm [52].

Mogamulizumab is a humanized IgG1 monoclonal antibody targeting the C-C chemokine receptor 4 (CCR4). CCR4 is expressed on lymphoma cells in T cell lymphomas including CTCL. CCR4 has been demonstrated to be overexpressed on the skin lesions in different stages of MF including patch, plaque, tumor MF and Sézary cells [49]. In a multicenter phase I-II clinical trial, patients with MF or SS were treated with IV infusion of mogamulizumab (0.1, 0.3, and 1.0 mg/kg) once weekly for 4 weeks followed by a 2-week observation with no dose-limiting toxicity and without reaching the maximum tolerated dose. In phase 2, patients were dosed with 1.0 mg/kg mogamulizumab with the same schedule for the first course followed by infusion every 2 weeks during subsequent courses until disease progression. Overall response rate was 36.8%, with 28.6% in the MF population and 47.1% in the SS population [53]. A phase II multi-center study showed similar efficacy in CTCL. Mogamulizumab was administered intravenously once per week for 8 weeks to 37 patients with relapsed CCR4-positive PTCL or CTCL. Overall response rate was 38% in patients with CTCL. The most common grade 3/4 treatment adverse effects were lymphocytopenia (81%, 73%), neutropenia (38%, 19%), and leukocytopenia (43%, 14%). The most common nonhematologic adverse effect was pyrexia (30%, grade 2 or lower). Lymphocytopenia was observed in 30 patients and was reported after the first dose in 26 of these patients. However, in 19 of the patients, lymphocyte counts were < 800/μL before the first dosing. Lymphocyte counts ultimately recovered to baseline or normal levels in all patients [54]. In the previously above mentioned MAVORIC trial, a phase III randomized, controlled study, treatment-emergent adverse events were more common with mogamulizumab in comparison to vorinostat, including infusion reactions and skin eruptions with 33.2% *compared to* 0.5% and 23.9% *vs.* 0.5%, respectively [45]. However, the study concluded that mogamulizumab significantly prolonged progression free survival compared with vorinostat (median 7.7 months vs. 3.1 months) [45]. The use of mogamulizumab has been associated with increased risk of acute graft versus host disease after allogeneic transplantation in Japanese patients with adult T-cell leukemia lymphoma. While the risk of acute graft versus host disease in patients with CTCL with allogeneic transplantation is unknown, the use of mogamulizumab in this population is discouraged [49].

Alemtuzumab is a humanized immunoglobulin G1 antibody against the CD52 molecule. CD52 is expressed on normal and malignant B and T lymphocytes [49]. Twenty-two patients with advanced MF and SS were involved in a phase II clinical trial [55]. The first dose was 3 mg, which was increased to 10 mg and then to 30 mg when infusion-related reactions were tolerated. The 30-mg dose was subsequently administered three times a week for up to 12 weeks. Treatment was stopped if the patient achieved complete response or met the criteria for progressive disease. The OR rate was 55%, with 32% of patients with a complete response and 23% with partial response [55]. Alemtuzumab was also reported to have activity in heavily treated CTCL in a study of seven patients with MF/SS and one with large-cell transformation of MF. Seven patients had disease refractory to multiple previous therapies. An overall response rate of 38% was reported; however, significant toxicity was observed with grade 3 or 4 cytopenias and significant infectious complications occurring in a majority of cases [56]. A recent study also reported that alemtuzumab could induce a long-term response, especially in patients with SS. Twenty-three patients with SS and 16 patients with MF were enrolled. All patients received alemtuzumab 30 mg 2-3 times per week for a median duration of 12 weeks with an overall response rate of 51% in all patients. The overall response rate was 70% in patients with SS, and 25% in patients with MF. Five SS patients and one MF patient remained relapse-free for greater than two years [57]. The most common side effects were infectious complications, including cytomegalovirus activation because of severe immunosuppression [49]. Alemtuzumab is not currently FDA-approved for CTCL. Due to the risk of opportunistic infection, patients receiving alemtuzumab should also receive anti-viral, anti-fungal, and PCP prophylaxis [49].

Combination Treatments

At early stages (IA, IB, IIA), MF is very responsive to the commonly used skin-directed treatments. However, skin-directed regimens can entail several adverse effects, such as the increased risk of skin cancer observed with PUVA or topical chemotherapy. Importantly, these therapeutic options can be ineffective to eradicate the malignant lymphoid cells in the peripheral blood, even in early disease [69]. Systemic treatments, such as interferon or oral retinoids can be used to address these problems. IFN is efficacious even in advanced disease, but its duration of response is short [70]. IFN-alfa used in conjunction with PUVA appears to improve complete response rate as compared to monotherapy [67]. Similarily, the use of a retinoids such as bexarotene combined with phototherapy also seems to have a synergistic effect. In a study of 69 MF plaque-stage patients who were treated with PUVA or oral retinoids plus PUVA, the response rates to treatment were equal, but the response was achieved with fewer PUVA treatments and lower cumulative UV-A dose in conjunction with systemic retinoids. Duration of remission was also longer when maintenance retinoids were used [71]. A retrospective study of 44 erythrodermic T4 MF patients suggested that a combination of TSEBT and ECP had a significant impact on progression-free survival and cause-specific survival as compared to TSEBT alone [72]. This synergistic effect does not apply to all forms of systemic therapy, however. A phase II clinical trial assessing the addition of IFN to bexarotene did not observe any difference in response rate to the expected response of bexarotene alone [73]. Bexarotene has also been found to be more effective in combination with ECP [34]. In patients with advanced stage disease and multiple poor prognostic factors, it is suggested that treatment with multimodality immunostimulatory therapy may experience higher clinical response rates and prolonged survival [74]. A large cohort study of 98 SS patients treated with at least 3 months of extracorporeal photopheresis and 1 or more systemic immunostimulatory agents observed high clinical response rates, with a complete response of 30% and a partial response of 45% [75].

Table 9-5. Combination treatment regimens

Skin directed and systemic therapies	Phototherapy + ECP Phototherapy + IFN alfa-2b or IFN gamma-1b Phototherapy + retinoid TSEBT + ECP
Systemic and systemic therapies	ECP + IFN alfa-2b or IFN gamma-1b ECP + retinoid ECP + retinoid + IFN alfa-2b or IFN gamma-1b Retinoid + IFN alfa-2b or IFN gamma-1b

CONCLUSION

The treatment modalities available for MF/SS widely range from skin-directed therapies to systemic therapies. When deciding upon the most appropriate treatment modality, a careful history, physical exam, and staging studies (and re-staging, if indicated) is paramount to choosing the most appropriate therapy. In general, patients with lower stage and skin-limited disease can be managed with escalating topical regimens or local phototherapy. As body-surface involvement increases, total body phototherapy may be more appropriate, with concurrent topical use for difficult to access areas. In patients with limited skin involvement but small foci of tumor, local radiation may be appropriate in conjunction with other skin-directed therapies.

In patients who have experienced inadequate responses to multiple skin-directed therapies, systemic treatments may be considered. Patients who also have >10% BSA involvement, folliculotropic disease, or large plaque or tumor involvement may also be considered for systemic therapy. Treatment with more conventional therapies, including IFN, methotrexate and bexarotene as well as novel and newer agents, such as CAR T-cell therapy, TTI-621, BNZ-1 or duvelisib may be considered, although access to the latter therapies may be limited in certain settings.

For refractory or relapsed disease, HDAC inhibitors (vorinostat, romidepsin), antibodies to CD30 (brentuximab), CD52 (alemtuzumab) or CCR4 (mogamulizumab) may also be appropriate. These treatments can have variable dosing schedules, and consideration must be made to patient access. For example, alemtuzumab is administered 3 times weekly, which may be more difficult for patient access compared mogamulizumab which is administered once everytwo weeks after the loading phase.

The unique challenges facing clinicians when treating MF/SS have resulted in significant research and development into increased options when considering treatment. Newer and novel therapies continue to develop, and will continue to add to the various treatment options available which will hopefully lead to increasingly tailored therapeutic regimens for patients' specific needs.

REFERENCES

[1] Jawed SI, Myskowski PL, Horwitz S, Moskowitz A, Querfeld C. Primary cutaneous T-cell lymphoma (mycosis fungoides and Sézary syndrome): Part II. Prognosis, management, and future directions. *Journal of the American Academy of Dermatology.* 2014;70 (2):223.e221-223.e217.

[2] Willemze R, Cerroni L, Kempf W, et al. The 2018 update of the WHO-EORTC classification for primary cutaneous lymphomas. *Blood.* 2019;133(16):1703-1714.

[3] Tarabadkar ES, Shinohara MM. Skin Directed Therapy in Cutaneous T-Cell Lymphoma. *Frontiers in oncology.* 2019;9:260.

[4] Zackheim HS, Kashani-Sabet M, Amin S. Topical corticosteroids for mycosis fungoides. Experience in 79 patients. *Arch Dermatol.* 1998;134(8):949-954.

[5] Lovgren M-L, Scarisbrick JJJCCO. Update on skin directed therapies in mycosis fungoides. 2018. 2018;8(1):7.

[6] Shipman AR, Scarisbrick J. New Treatment Options for Mycosis Fungoides. *Indian journal of dermatology.* 2016;61(1):119.

[7] Rook AH, Gelfand JM, Wysocka M, et al. Topical resiquimod can induce disease regression and enhance T-cell effector functions in cutaneous T-cell lymphoma. *Blood.* 2015;126(12):1452-1461.

[8] Lessin SR, Duvic M, Guitart J, et al. Topical chemotherapy in cutaneous T-cell lymphoma: positive results of a randomized, controlled, multicenter trial testing the efficacy and safety of a novel mechlorethamine, 0.02%, gel in mycosis fungoides. *JAMA dermatology.* 2013;149(1):25-32.

[9] Breneman D, Duvic M, Kuzel T, Yocum R, Truglia J, Stevens VJ. Phase 1 and 2 trial of bexarotene gel for skin-directed treatment of patients with cutaneous T-cell lymphoma. *Arch Dermatol.* 2002;138(3):325-332.

[10] Besner Morin C, Roberge D, Turchin I, Petrogiannis-Haliotis T, Popradi G, Pehr K. Tazarotene 0.1% Cream as Monotherapy for Early-

Stage Cutaneous T-Cell Lymphoma. *Journal of cutaneous medicine and surgery.* 2016;20(3):244-248.

[11] Apisarnthanarax N, Talpur R, Ward S, Ni X, Kim HW, Duvic M. Tazarotene 0.1% gel for refractory mycosis fungoides lesions: an open-label pilot study. *J Am Acad Dermatol.* 2004;50(4):600-607.

[12] Zackheim HS, Epstein EH, Jr., Crain WR. Topical carmustine (BCNU) for cutaneous T cell lymphoma: a 15-year experience in 143 patients. *J Am Acad Dermatol.* 1990;22(5 Pt 1):802-810.

[13] Rallis E, Economidi A, Verros C, Papadakis P. Successful treatment of patch type mycosis fungoides with tacrolimus ointment 0.1%. *Journal of drugs in dermatology: JDD.* 2006;5(9):906-907.

[14] Siegfried EC, Jaworski JC, Hebert AA. Topical calcineurin inhibitors and lymphoma risk: evidence update with implications for daily practice. *American journal of clinical dermatology.* 2013;14(3):163-178.

[15] Vaqué JP, Gómez-López G, Monsálvez V, et al. PLCG1 mutations in cutaneous T-cell lymphomas. *Blood.* 2014;123(13):2034-2043.

[16] Patraquim C, Gomes MM, Garcez C, et al. Childhood Hypopigmented Mycosis Fungoides: A Rare Diagnosis. *Case reports in pediatrics.* 2016;2016:8564389.

[17] Ortiz-Romero P, Maronas-Jiménez L, Muniesa C, et al. Interim analysis of phase II clinical trial PIMTOMF (Topical pimecrolimus in early MF) EUDRA CT 2014-001377-1. In. 3rd World Conference of Cutaneous Lymphomas: Hospital Universitario 12 de Octubre, Instituto de Investigación Madrid. Hospital Clinic de Barcelona. Universitat de Barcelona. Idibaps Hospital Universitari de Bellvitge, Barcelona. Hospital Nuestra Señora de la Candelaria. Santa Cruz de Tenerife. IVO, Valencia. Hospital del Mar. Barcelona. Instituto de Investigación Sanitaria Puerta de Hierro-Majadahonda. Madrid; 2016.

[18] Abędź N, Pawliczak R. Efficacy and safety of topical calcineurin inhibitors for the treatment of atopic dermatitis: meta-analysis of randomized clinical trials. *Postepy dermatologii i alergologii.* 2019;36(6):752-759.

[19] Long CC, Finlay AY. The finger-tip unit--a new practical measure. *Clinical and experimental dermatology.* 1991;16(6):444-447.

[20] Specht L, Dabaja B, Illidge T, Wilson LD, Hoppe RT. Modern Radiation Therapy for Primary Cutaneous Lymphomas: Field and Dose Guidelines From the International Lymphoma Radiation Oncology Group. *International Journal of Radiation Oncology*Biology*Physics.* 2015;92(1):32-39.

[21] Navi D, Riaz N, Levin YS, Sullivan NC, Kim YH, Hoppe RT. The Stanford University experience with conventional-dose, total skin electron-beam therapy in the treatment of generalized patch or plaque (T2) and tumor (T3) mycosis fungoides. *Arch Dermatol.* 2011;147(5):561-567.

[22] Hodak E, Pavlovsky L. Phototherapy of Mycosis Fungoides. *Dermatologic Clinics.* 2015;33(4):697-702.

[23] Querfeld C, Rosen ST, Kuzel TM, et al. Long-term follow-up of patients with early-stage cutaneous T-cell lymphoma who achieved complete remission with psoralen plus UV-A monotherapy. *Arch Dermatol.* 2005;141(3):305-311.

[24] Scarfò I, Frigault MJ, Maus MV. CAR-Based Approaches to Cutaneous T-Cell Lymphoma. *Frontiers in oncology.* 2019;9:259.

[25] Johnson LDS, Banerjee S, Kruglov O, et al. Targeting CD47 in Sézary syndrome with SIRPαFc. *Blood advances.* 2019;3(7):1145-1153.

[26] Bagot M, Porcu P, Marie-Cardine A, et al. IPH4102, a first-in-class anti-KIR3DL2 monoclonal antibody, in patients with relapsed or refractory cutaneous T-cell lymphoma: an international, first-in-human, open-label, phase 1 trial. *The Lancet Oncology.* 2019;20(8):1160-1170.

[27] Seto AG, Beatty X, Lynch JM, et al. Cobomarsen, an oligonucleotide inhibitor of miR-155, co-ordinately regulates multiple survival pathways to reduce cellular proliferation and survival in cutaneous T-cell lymphoma. *British journal of haematology.* 2018;183(3):428-444.

[28] Khodadoust MS, Rook AH, Porcu P, et al. Pembrolizumab in Relapsed and Refractory Mycosis Fungoides and Sézary Syndrome: A Multicenter Phase II Study. *Journal of clinical oncology: official*

journal of the American Society of Clinical Oncology. 2020;38(1):20-28.

[29] Frankel AE, Woo JH, Ahn C, et al. Resimmune, an anti-CD3ε recombinant immunotoxin, induces durable remissions in patients with cutaneous T-cell lymphoma. *Haematologica.* 2015;100(6):794-800.

[30] Querfeld C, William BM, Brammer JE, et al. Bnz-1, a Selective γ-Chain Cytokine Inhibitor Has Clinical Activity in Patients with Cutaneous T Cell Lymphoma By Selectively Blocking IL-2, IL-15 and IL-9 Signaling: Results of a Multicenter, Open-Label Phase 1 Trial. *Blood.* 2019;134(Supplement_1):1557-1557.

[31] Horwitz SM, Koch R, Porcu P, et al. Activity of the PI3K-δ,γ inhibitor duvelisib in a phase 1 trial and preclinical models of T-cell lymphoma. *Blood.* 2018;131(8):888-898.

[32] Cheeley J, Sahn RE, DeLong LK, Parker SR. Acitretin for the treatment of cutaneous T-cell lymphoma. *J Am Acad Dermatol.* 2013;68(2):247-254.

[33] Zhang C, Duvic M. Treatment of cutaneous T-cell lymphoma with retinoids. *Dermatologic therapy.* 2006;19(5):264-271.

[34] Zhang C, Duvic M. Retinoids: therapeutic applications and mechanisms of action in cutaneous T-cell lymphoma. *Dermatologic therapy.* 2003;16(4):322-330.

[35] Talpur R, Ward S, Apisarnthanarax N, Breuer-Mcham J, Duvic M. Optimizing bexarotene therapy for cutaneous T-cell lymphoma. *J Am Acad Dermatol.* 2002;47(5):672-684.

[36] Zackheim HS, Kashani-Sabet M, Hwang ST. Low-dose methotrexate to treat erythrodermic cutaneous T-cell lymphoma: results in twenty-nine patients. *J Am Acad Dermatol.* 1996;34(4):626-631.

[37] Zackheim HS, Kashani-Sabet M, McMillan A. Low-dose methotrexate to treat mycosis fungoides: a retrospective study in 69 patients. *J Am Acad Dermatol.* 2003;49(5):873-878.

[38] Olsen EA. Interferon in the treatment of cutaneous T-cell lymphoma. *Dermatologic therapy.* 2003;16(4):311-321.

[39] Olsen EA, Rosen ST, Vollmer RT, et al. Interferon alfa-2a in the treatment of cutaneous T cell lymphoma. *J Am Acad Dermatol.* 1989;20(3):395-407.

[40] Atilla E, Atilla PA, Bozdag SC, et al. Extracorporeal photochemotherapy in mycosis fungoides. *Transfusion clinique et biologique: journal de la Societe francaise de transfusion sanguine.* 2017;24(4):454-457.

[41] Knobler R, Duvic M, Querfeld C, et al. Long-term follow-up and survival of cutaneous T-cell lymphoma patients treated with extracorporeal photopheresis. *Photodermatology, photoimmunology & photomedicine.* 2012;28(5):250-257.

[42] Olsen EA, Whittaker S, Kim YH, et al. Clinical end points and response criteria in mycosis fungoides and Sézary syndrome: a consensus statement of the International Society for Cutaneous Lymphomas, the United States Cutaneous Lymphoma Consortium, and the Cutaneous Lymphoma Task Force of the European Organisation for Research and Treatment of Cancer. *Journal of clinical oncology: official journal of the American Society of Clinical Oncology.* 2011;29(18):2598-2607.

[43] Olsen EA, Kim YH, Kuzel TM, et al. Phase IIb multicenter trial of vorinostat in patients with persistent, progressive, or treatment refractory cutaneous T-cell lymphoma. *Journal of clinical oncology: official journal of the American Society of Clinical Oncology.* 2007;25(21):3109-3115.

[44] Duvic M, Olsen EA, Breneman D, et al. Evaluation of the long-term tolerability and clinical benefit of vorinostat in patients with advanced cutaneous T-cell lymphoma. *Clinical lymphoma & myeloma.* 2009;9(6):412-416.

[45] Kim YH, Bagot M, Pinter-Brown L, et al. Mogamulizumab versus vorinostat in previously treated cutaneous T-cell lymphoma (MAVORIC): an international, open-label, randomised, controlled phase 3 trial. *The Lancet Oncology.* 2018;19(9):1192-1204.

[46] Whittaker SJ, Demierre MF, Kim EJ, et al. Final results from a multicenter, international, pivotal study of romidepsin in refractory

cutaneous T-cell lymphoma. *Journal of clinical oncology: official journal of the American Society of Clinical Oncology.* 2010;28(29):4485-4491.

[47] Piekarz RL, Frye R, Turner M, et al. Phase II multi-institutional trial of the histone deacetylase inhibitor romidepsin as monotherapy for patients with cutaneous T-cell lymphoma. *Journal of clinical oncology: official journal of the American Society of Clinical Oncology.* 2009;27(32):5410-5417.

[48] Kim YH, Demierre MF, Kim EJ, et al. Clinically meaningful reduction in pruritus in patients with cutaneous T-cell lymphoma treated with romidepsin. *Leukemia & lymphoma.* 2013;54(2):284-289.

[49] Alpdogan O, Kartan S, Johnson W, Sokol K, Porcu PJCCO. Systemic therapy of cutaneous T-cell lymphoma (CTCL). *2019.* 2019;8(1):10.

[50] Kim YH, Tavallaee M, Sundram U, et al. Phase II Investigator-Initiated Study of Brentuximab Vedotin in Mycosis Fungoides and Sézary Syndrome with Variable CD30 Expression Level: A Multi-Institution Collaborative Project. *Journal of clinical oncology: official journal of the American Society of Clinical Oncology.* 2015;33(32):3750-3758.

[51] Duvic M, Tetzlaff MT, Gangar P, Clos AL, Sui D, Talpur R. Results of a Phase II Trial of Brentuximab Vedotin for CD30+ Cutaneous T-Cell Lymphoma and Lymphomatoid Papulosis. *Journal of clinical oncology: official journal of the American Society of Clinical Oncology.* 2015;33(32):3759-3765.

[52] Prince HM, Kim YH, Horwitz SM, et al. Brentuximab vedotin or physician's choice in CD30-positive cutaneous T-cell lymphoma (ALCANZA): an international, open-label, randomised, phase 3, multicentre trial. *Lancet (London, England).* 2017;390(10094):555-566.

[53] Duvic M, Pinter-Brown LC, Foss FM, et al. Phase 1/2 study of mogamulizumab, a defucosylated anti-CCR4 antibody, in previously treated patients with cutaneous T-cell lymphoma. *Blood.* 2015;125(12):1883-1889.

[54] Ogura M, Ishida T, Hatake K, et al. Multicenter phase II study of mogamulizumab (KW-0761), a defucosylated anti-cc chemokine receptor 4 antibody, in patients with relapsed peripheral T-cell lymphoma and cutaneous T-cell lymphoma. *Journal of clinical oncology: official journal of the American Society of Clinical Oncology.* 2014;32(11):1157-1163.

[55] Lundin J, Hagberg H, Repp R, et al. Phase 2 study of alemtuzumab (anti-CD52 monoclonal antibody) in patients with advanced mycosis fungoides/Sézary syndrome. *Blood.* 2003;101(11):4267-4272.

[56] Kennedy GA, Seymour JF, Wolf M, et al. Treatment of patients with advanced mycosis fungoides and Sézary syndrome with alemtuzumab. *European journal of haematology.* 2003;71(4):250-256.

[57] de Masson A, Guitera P, Brice P, et al. Long-term efficacy and safety of alemtuzumab in advanced primary cutaneous T-cell lymphomas. *The British journal of dermatology.* 2014;170(3):720-724.

[58] Photiou L, van der Weyden C, McCormack C, Miles Prince H. Systemic Treatment Options for Advanced-Stage Mycosis Fungoides and Sézary Syndrome. *Current Oncology Reports.* 2018;20(4):32.

[59] Coors EA, von den Driesch P. Treatment of erythrodermic cutaneous T-cell lymphoma with intermittent chlorambucil and fluocortolone therapy. *The British journal of dermatology.* 2000;143(1):127-131.

[60] Duvic M. Choosing a systemic treatment for advanced stage cutaneous T-cell lymphoma: mycosis fungoides and Sézary syndrome. *Hematology.* 2015;2015(1):529-544.

[61] Greiner D, Olsen EA, Petroni G. Pentostatin (2'-deoxycoformycin) in the treatment of cutaneous T-cell lymphoma. *J Am Acad Dermatol.* 1997;36(6 Pt 1):950-955.

[62] Foss FM. Activity of pentostatin (Nipent) in cutaneous T-cell lymphoma: single-agent and combination studies. *Seminars in oncology.* 2000;27(2 Suppl 5):58-63.

[63] Querfeld C, Rosen ST, Guitart J, et al. Multicenter phase II trial of temozolomide in mycosis fungoides/Sézary syndrome: correlation with O^6-methylguanine-DNA methyltransferase and mismatch repair

proteins. *Clinical cancer research: an official journal of the American Association for Cancer Research.* 2011;17(17):5748-5754.

[64] Bird TG, Whittaker S, Wain EM, Child F, Morris SL. Temozolomide for central nervous system involvement in mycosis fungoides. *International journal of dermatology.* 2016;55(7):751-756.

[65] Zinzani PL, Musuraca G, Tani M, et al. Phase II trial of proteasome inhibitor bortezomib in patients with relapsed or refractory cutaneous T-cell lymphoma. *Journal of clinical oncology: official journal of the American Society of Clinical Oncology.* 2007;25(27):4293-4297.

[66] Duvic M, Talpur R, Wen S, Kurzrock R, David CL, Apisarnthanarax N. Phase II evaluation of gemcitabine monotherapy for cutaneous T-cell lymphoma. *Clinical lymphoma & myeloma.* 2006;7(1):51-58.

[67] Horwitz SM, Kim YH, Foss F, et al. Identification of an active, well-tolerated dose of pralatrexate in patients with relapsed or refractory cutaneous T-cell lymphoma. *Blood.* 2012;119(18):4115-4122.

[68] Chung CG, Poligone B. Cutaneous T cell Lymphoma: an Update on Pathogenesis and Systemic Therapy. *Current hematologic malignancy reports.* 2015;10(4):468-476.

[69] Rupoli S, Goteri G, Pulini S, et al. Long-term experience with low-dose interferon-alpha and PUVA in the management of early mycosis fungoides. *European journal of haematology.* 2005;75(2):136-145.

[70] Stadler R, Otte HG, Luger T, et al. Prospective randomized multicenter clinical trial on the use of interferon -2a plus acitretin versus interferon -2a plus PUVA in patients with cutaneous T-cell lymphoma stages I and II. *Blood.* 1998;92(10):3578-3581.

[71] McGinnis KS, Shapiro M, Vittorio CC, Rook AH, Junkins-Hopkins JM. Psoralen plus long-wave UV-A (PUVA) and bexarotene therapy: An effective and synergistic combined adjunct to therapy for patients with advanced cutaneous T-cell lymphoma. *Arch Dermatol.* 2003;139(6):771-775.

[72] Wilson LD, Jones GW, Kim D, et al. Experience with total skin electron beam therapy in combination with extracorporeal photopheresis in the management of patients with erythrodermic (T4) mycosis fungoides. *J Am Acad Dermatol.* 2000;43(1 Pt 1):54-60.

[73] Straus DJ, Duvic M, Kuzel T, et al. Results of a phase II trial of oral bexarotene (Targretin) combined with interferon alfa-2b (Intron-A) for patients with cutaneous T-cell lymphoma. *Cancer.* 2007;109(9):1799-1803.

[74] Suchin KR, Cucchiara AJ, Gottleib SL, et al. Treatment of cutaneous T-cell lymphoma with combined immunomodulatory therapy: a 14-year experience at a single institution. *Arch Dermatol.* 2002;138(8):1054-1060.

[75] Raphael BA, Shin DB, Suchin KR, et al. High clinical response rate of Sézary syndrome to immunomodulatory therapies: prognostic markers of response. *Arch Dermatol.* 2011;147(12):1410-1415.

In: Mycosis Fungoides and Sézary Syndrome ISBN: 978-1-68507-093-9
Editors: X. Zhang and L. Sokol

Chapter 10

STAGING AND PROGNOSIS OF MYCOSIS FUNGOIDES

Kerry Hennessy, MD, Nicole Nagrani, MD and Lucia Seminario-Vidal[1,*], MD, PhD

[1]Department of Dermatology and Cutaneous Surgery, University of South Florida, Tampa, FL, USA

[2]Department of Cutaneous Oncology, H. Lee Moffitt Cancer Center and Research Institute, Tampa, FL, USA

INTRODUCTION

Mycosis fungoides (MF) was originally described by Jean Louis Alibert in 1806 as 'pian fungoide.' This term later evolved into mycosis fungoides as the lesions often resemble mushrooms. Over time, as nomenclature changed, so did knowledge of the disease and stratification thereof. Clinical staging has become of paramount importance in not only identifying the

* Corresponding Author's Email: luciasem@usf.edu.

appropriate treatment for MF but also to determine prognosis [1]. Herein, we discuss the staging systems used for MF and their role in prognosis.

Staging

The staging of mycosis fungoides (MF) has changed over time with advances in knowledge of the disease. Classification historically included all types of cutaneous T-cell lymphomas (CTCLs) but today has evolved into separate categories that also reflect the level of blood involvement.

MF usually follows a classic pattern of evolution from patches to plaques to tumors and erythroderma. However, it is important to note that patients may often seem to skip one of these stages, present with various types of lesions, or go undiagnosed in the early stages when these clinical lesions are present [1].

The natural history of the disease begins with patches that initially appear in affected subjects and are defined as any lesion without significant induration or elevation above the surrounding skin. In the next stage, plaques (any lesion that is elevated or indurated compared to the surrounding skin surface) develop. As the disease progresses, patients may grow tumors– any solid or nodular lesions greater than or equal to one centimeter in diameter, demonstrating vertical growth or infiltration into the underlying skin [2].

In the final stage of skin involvement, erythroderma is possible. Many patients will actually present erythrodermic skipping the other stages of disease and presenting a diagnostic challenge for physicians. In CTCL, erythroderma is considered as erythema equaling or greater than 80% of body surface area (BSA) [2].

Disease severity can be assessed utilizing the modified severity weighted assessment tool, also known as the mSWAT. This serves as an objective global scoring system to determine overall disease burden by incorporating the percentage of body surface involvement by each type of body lesion (patch/plaque/tumor). The palmar surface of the hand and the fingers is considered 1% BSA for calculation purposes. Note that this is the patient's hand and therefore will change with them as they grow and age [3].

Equation and Table 10-1 showing the mSWAT scoring system are depicted below:

Equation 1, mSWAT**:** sum of BSA of each body region multiplied by a weighting factor for the type of lesion.

mSWAT = (subtotal BSA patch ×1) + (subtotal BSA plaque ×2) + (subtotal BSA tumor × 4)

In addition to scoring based on clinical lesions, a TNMB classification system is used for the categorization of disease in MF. In this case, tumor represents skin involvement, nodes for affected lymph nodes (LN), metastasis as visceral involvement and blood for level of tumor burden in the blood.

Table 10-1. mSWAT

Body Region (%BSA)	**Patch**	**Plaque**	**Tumor**
Head (7%)			
Neck (2%)			
Anterior trunk (13%)			
Arms (8%)			
Forearms (6%)			
Hands (5%)			
Posterior trunk (13%)			
Buttocks (5%)			
Thighs (19%)			
Legs (14%)			
Feet (7%)			
Groin (1%)			
Subtotal BSA			
Weighting Factor	×1	×2	×4
Subtotal BSA x weighting factor			
mSWAT score= summation of each of the columns above			

Table 10-2. TNMB Classification as adapted from the NCCN Guidelines

TNMB		**TNMB Classification and Staging of Mycosis Fungoides and Sézary Syndrome (SS)**
Skin	T1	Limited patches, papules and/or plaques covering <10% BSA
	T2	Patches, papules and/or plaques covering ≥10% BSA
	T2a	Patch phase only
	T2b	Plaque +/- patch
	T3	One or more tumors
	T4	Confluent erythema ≥80% BSA
Node	N0	No clinically abnormal LNs
	N1	Abnormal LNs; histopathologic Dutch Grade 1 or NCI LN 0-2
	N2	Abnormal LNs; histopathologic Dutch Grade 2 or NCI LN 3
	N3	Abnormal LNs; histopathologic Dutch Grade 3-4 or NCI LN 4
	NX	Abnormal LNs without histologic confirmation
Visceral	M0	No visceral organ involvement
	M1	Viscera involvement (requiring pathological confirmation and organ specified)
	MX	Abnormal visceral site without histological confirmation
Blood	B0	Absence of significant blood involvement: ≤5% of peripheral blood lymphocytes or <250/μL are atypical (Sézary) cells OR <15% CD4+/CD26- or CD4+/CD7- cells of total lymphocytes
	B1	Low blood tumor burden: >5% of peripheral blood lymphocytes are atypical cells OR ≥15% CD4+CD26- or CD4+CD7- of total lymphocytes but do not meet the criteria of B0 or B2
	B2	High blood tumor burden: ≥1000/μL atypical cells determined by cytopathology OR ≥1000 CD4+CD26- or CD4+CD7- cells/μL or other abnormal subset of T lymphocytes by flow cytometry with clone in blood same as that in the skin. Other criteria for CD4+ MF/SS include CD4+/CD7- cells ≥40% and CD4+CD26- cells ≥30%

Table 10-2 is adapted from the National Comprehensive Cancer Network (NCCN) guidelines [2].

Lymph node classification of MF includes the National Cancer Institute lymph node grading system (NCI-LN) as well as the Dutch criteria for lymph nodes [4]. These are represented by Tables 10-3 and 10-4 respectively.

The blood classification of MF/SS has yet to be standardized. A systematic review by Scarisbrick et al. in 2018 reported that there is no objective blood staging system according to flow cytometry in the literature. The authors then go on to compare proposed blood staging systems [5].

Table 10-3. National Cancer Institute - Lymph Nodes (NCI-LN) grade system

NCI-LN	
LN 0	No atypical lymphocytes
LN 1	Occasional and isolated atypical lymphocytes, not arranged in clusters
LN 2	Many atypical lymphocytes OR in 3-6 cell clusters
LN 3	Aggregates of atypical lymphocytes with nodal architecture preserved
LN 4	Partial/complete effacement of nodal architecture by atypical lymphocytes or frankly neoplastic cells

Table 10-4. Dutch criteria for lymph nodes

Dutch Grade System	
Grade 1	Dermatopathic lymphadenopathy (DL)
Grade 2	Early involvement by MF, (presence of cerebriform nuclei > 7.5 micrometers (μm)
Grade 3	Partial effacement of lymph node architecture; many atypical cerebriform mononuclear cells (CMCs)
Grade 4	Complete effacement of lymph node architecture

Table 10-5. Blood staging by flow cytometry

Author	B0	B1	B2
Vonderheid et al. 2018 [6]	<30% CD4+CD26-	≥30% CD4+CD26- and <1000/μL	CD4+CD26- ≥1000/μL
NCCN Guidelines 2021 [2]	Absence of significant blood involvement: ≤5% of peripheral blood lymphocytes or <250/μL are atypical (Sézary) cells OR <15% CD4+CD26- or CD4+CD7- cells of total lymphocytes	Low blood tumor burden: >5% of peripheral blood lymphocytes are atypical cells OR ≥15% CD4+CD26- or CD4+CD7- of total lymphocytes but do not meet the criteria of B0 or B2	High blood tumor burden: ≥1000/μL atypical cells determined by cytopathology OR ≥1000 CD4+CD26- or CD4+CD7- cells/μL or other abnormal subset of T lymphocytes by flow cytometry with clone in blood same as that in the skin Other criteria for CD4+ MF/SS include CD4+CD7- cells ≥40% and CD4+CD26- cells ≥30%
PROCLIPI [7]	<250/μL CD4+CD7- or CD4+CD26- cells/μL	250/μL to <1000/μL CD4+CD7- or CD4+CD26- cells/μL	≥1000/μL CD4+CD7- or CD4+CD26- cells/μL (or other aberrant phenotype) + evidence of a relevant T-cell clone in blood that is same as that in the skin

One such classification, proposed by Vonderheid et al. in 2018, categorizes B0 as <30% CD4+CD26- and <1000/μL with B1 being the reverse (≥30% CD4+CD26- and <1000/μL). B2 is then defined as CD4+CD26- ≥1000/μL [6]. The NCCN guidelines and PROCLIPI offer two other definitions of blood involvement as compared in the table below (Table 10-5, adapted from Scarisbrick et al.) [5].

Using the aforementioned components, a clinical staging for MF and SS can be constructed, allowing for straightforward disease classification. Table 10-6 is adapted from the NCCN guidelines and reflects this useful system [2].

PROGNOSIS

Mycosis Fungoides has a variable clinical presentation, and differentiation from benign inflammatory skin diseases such as eczema or psoriasis can be difficult.

Table 10-6. Clinical Staging of MF and SS

Clinical Stage	T (Skin)	N (Nodes)	M (Visceral)	B (Blood)
IA	T1 (<10% BSA)	N0	M0	B0-1
IB	T2 (≥10% but < 80% BSA)	N0	M0	B0-1
IIA	T1-2	N1-2	M0	B0-1
IIB	T3 (≥1 tumor)	N0-2	M0	B0-1
IIIA	T4 (erythema ≥80% BSA)	N0-2	M0	B0
IIIB	T4 (erythema ≥80% BSA)	N0-2	M0	B1
IVA1	T1-4	N0-2	M0	B2
IVA2	T1-4	N3	M0	B0-2
IVB	T1-4	N0-3	M1	B0-2

Diagnostic delay of a median duration of 36 months was found in 85.6% of patients from the onset of lesions to the diagnosis of early-stage MF [7]. Failure to correctly diagnose CTCL can lead to inappropriate therapy and a delay in therapeutic management, therefore affecting prognosis.

For this reason, many efforts have been made to identify prognostic factors to guide management and predict survival outcomes.

The most important prognostic factor in mycosis fungoides is the TNMB stage. Additional risk factors for disease progression include the overall stage, type of skin involvement, presence of extracutaneous disease, blood involvement, age at presentation, elevated lactate dehydrogenase, and presence of large cell transformation [7]. Of these risk factors, the age of the patient (greater than 60), the T classification, and the presence of extracutaneous disease have shown independent clinical prognostic value [8, 9]. The initial T classification (T1, T2, T3, and T4) has also been found to correlate with progression to more advanced disease, worse clinical stage, development of extracutaneous disease and even death due to MF [8]. Although N/M/B staging, age, and male sex are predictors of poor survival, these factors were not associated with disease progression [9].

The degree of skin involvement and overall clinical stage have consistently shown a positive correlation with progressive disease and decreased survival. Individuals with limited patch/plaque disease have a good prognosis, without altered life expectancy compared to age/race/sex-matched control population [10]. Moreover, those with purely cutaneous patch disease have an increased overall survival and decreased progression risk as compared to those with plaque disease [9]. Widespread disease involvement, as with tumor stage and erythroderma, is associated with a worse prognosis. As expected, the development of Sézary syndrome is associated with a poorer prognosis than those solely with erythroderma [11].

Based on the pooled data of 6,279 patients with MF (stage IA to IVB), Mourad et al. estimated the stage-specific 5-year overall survival rates reflecting the median, best and worst case prognoses (Fig. 10-1) [12].

In another study, data from 525 patients with MF/SS was used to calculate stage-specific survival rates of five to 15 years with results ranging from 96% to 73% for stage IA, 75% to 46% for stage IB/IIA, 44% to 15% for stage IIB/III, and 27% to 10% for stage IV [8].

Data from the Cutaneous Lymphoma International Consortium Study (CLIC) meta-analysis of 1,275 patients with advanced MF (stage IIA to IV) showed decreased survival with increasing stage of disease. This study further identified four risk factors with independent prognostic significance: LDH, large cell transformation, increasing age, and Stage IV disease. A prognostic index model including these four variables was used to stratify risk groups and their associated survival outcomes; low risk (zero to one variable), intermediate risk (two variables), and high risk (three to four variables), with 5-year predicted overall survival (OS) rates of 67.8%, 43.5%, and 27.6%, respectively [13].

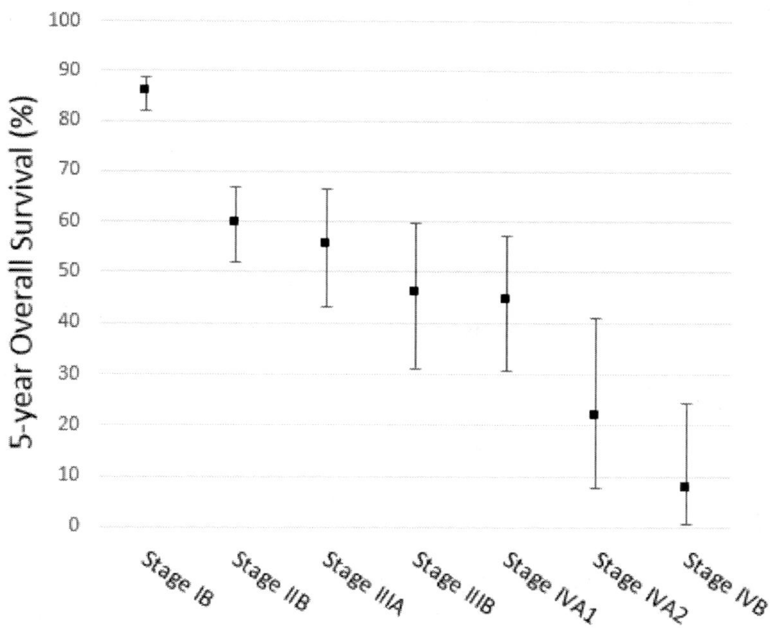

Figure 10-1. Stage-specific 5-year survival rate [12].

Additional efforts to formulate prognostic indices were made using the cutaneous lymphoma international prognostic index (CLIPi). This retrospective analysis of 1,502 patients identified adverse prognostic factors for early-stage MF (IA to IIA) which included male gender, age >60, plaques, folliculotropic disease, and stage N1/Nx. The study also identified adverse prognostic indicators for advanced (IIB to IVB) stage MF and SS—these included male gender, age >60, stages B1/B2, N2/3, and visceral involvement. These variables were then used to define three prognostic groups for both early and advanced stage MF: 0 - 1 (low risk), 2 (intermediate risk), and 3 - 5 factors (high risk). Patients with early-stage MF had estimated 10-year OS rates of 90.3% (low risk), 76.2% (intermediate risk) and 48.9% (high risk). In the late-stage model, OS rates were 53.2% in the low-risk category, 19.8% in the intermediate and 15.0% in the high-risk group [14]. These data were then validated using 1,202 patients from an independent institution which showed similar OS rates. Nevertheless, data assessing prognostic risk in MF/SS is limited and further prospective trials are warranted to verify the accuracy of prognostic indices and projected survival outcomes.

SUMMARY

Staging is crucial in the diagnosis of Mycosis fungoides since this classification not only guides management but is highly indicative of prognosis. The standard staging of MF is determined by the TNMB classification system which includes the grade of skin (T), lymph node (N),visceral (M) and blood (B) involvement. The prognosis of MF varies depending upon multiple factors, however, advanced clinical stages are most often directly correlated with disease progression and decreased survival.

REFERENCES

[1] Bolognia, J., Jorizzo, J. and Schaffer, J. History, in *Dermatology*, 2018, Elsevier: Philadelphia. p. 2127.

[2] Mehta-Shah, N. et al. *NCCN Guidelines Insights: Primary Cutaneous Lymphomas,* Version 2.2020. 2020. 18(5): p. 522.

[3] Scarisbrick, J. J. Skin Scoring for Mycosis Fungoides and Sézary Syndrome, in *Measuring the Skin*. 2016, Springer International Publishing: Cham. p. 1 - 11.

[4] Institute, N. C., *TNM Data v1.0.*

[5] Scarisbrick, J. J. et al. Blood classification and blood response criteria in mycosis fungoides and Sézary syndrome using flow cytometry: Recommendations from the EORTC cutaneous lymphoma task force. *Eur. J. Cancer*, 2018. 93: p. 47 - 56.

[6] Vonderheid, E. C. and Hou, J. S. CD4+CD26− lymphocytes are useful to assess blood involvement and define B ratings in cutaneous T cell lymphoma. 2018. Great Britain: Informa Healthcare.

[7] Scarisbrick, J. J. et al. The PROCLIPI international registry of early-stage mycosis fungoides identifies substantial diagnostic delay in most patients. *Br. J. Dermatol.,* 2019. 181(2): p. 350 - 357.

[8] Kim, Y. H. et al. Long-term outcome of 525 patients with mycosis fungoides and Sézary syndrome: Clinical prognostic factors and risk for disease progression. *Arch. Dermatol.*, 2003. 139(7): p. 857 - 66.

[9] Agar, N. S. et al. Survival outcomes and prognostic factors in mycosis fungoides/Sézary syndrome: Validation of the revised International Society for Cutaneous Lymphomas/European Organisation for Research and Treatment of Cancer staging proposal. *J. Clin. Oncol.,* 2010. 28(31): p. 4730 - 9.

[10] Kim, Y. H. et al. Clinical stage IA (limited patch and plaque) mycosis fungoides. A long-term outcome analysis. *Arch. Dermatol.,* 1996. 132(11): p. 1309 - 13.

[11] Kim, Y. H. et al. Prognostic factors in erythrodermic mycosis fungoides and the Sézary syndrome. *Arch. Dermatol.,* 1995. 131(9): p. 1003 - 8.

[12] Mourad, A. and Gniadecki, R. Overall Survival in Mycosis Fungoides: A Systematic Review and Meta-Analysis. *J. Invest. Dermatol.*, 2020. 140(2): p. 495 - 497 e5.

[13] Scarisbrick, J. J. et al. Cutaneous Lymphoma International Consortium Study of Outcome in Advanced Stages of Mycosis Fungoides and Sézary Syndrome: Effect of Specific Prognostic Markers on Survival and Development of a Prognostic Model. *J. Clin. Oncol.*, 2015. 33(32): p. 3766 - 73.

[14] Benton, E. C. et al. A cutaneous lymphoma international prognostic index (CLIPi) for mycosis fungoides and Sézary syndrome. *Eur. J. Cancer,* 2013. 49(13): p. 2859 - 68.

In: Mycosis Fungoides and Sézary Syndrome ISBN: 978-1-68507-093-9
Editors: X. Zhang and L. Sokol

Chapter 11

Clinical Features, Systemic Treatment, and Prognosis of Sézary Syndrome

Ashley Rose, MD and Lubomir Sokol*, MD, PhD
Department of Malignant Hematology,
H. Lee Moffitt Cancer Center and Research Institute, Tampa, FL, USA

Introduction

Sézary syndrome (SS) is a rare, leukemic form of cutaneous T-cell lymphoma, with circulating malignant T-cells in the blood that typically match the clone found in the skin. The term "Sézary Syndrome" was coined by French Dermatologist, Dr. Albert Sézary, in the late 1930's who described patients presenting with erythroderma and very large abnormal cells in the blood [1]. SS may evolve from patch/plaque or erythrodermic mycosis fungoides or may present de novo. Patients with SS are typically more symptomatic and overall have more aggressive disease and shorter expected survival compared to those with MF.

---

* Corresponding Author's Email: Lubomir.Sokol@moffitt.org

CLINICAL FEATURES

Sézary syndrome typically affects older adults with median age >60 years and with a male: female ratio of 2:1 [2]. The estimated incidence of SS is 0.8 cases per million persons per year [2]. The classic presentation is defined by the triad of erythroderma, peripheral lymphadenopathy, and leukemic blood involvement [3].

Patients with SS commonly present with diffuse erythroderma which may be exfoliative, scaly, indurated, or resemble livido reticularis [4]. Typically, the disease involves >80% body surface area (BSA) which meets the definition of erythroderma. This is considered skin stage T4 by Mycosis Fungoides Cooperative Group and International Society for Cutaneous Lymphomas (ISCL) and the cutaneous lymphoma task force of the European Organization of Research and Treatment of Cancer (EORTC) [5, 6]. Blood involvement with Sézary cells usually manifests with a high tumor burden with >1,000/μL, which is consistent with stage B2 [5]. Additional parameters consistent with stage B2 using flow cytometry include the presence of immunophenotypically abnormal T cells such CD4+/CD26- or CD4+/CD7- populations comprising 30% or 40% of total lymphocytes in peripheral blood, respectively. Severe pruritis may be present months to years prior to diagnosis [4]. Pruritis is the most common and often most debilitating symptom associated with SS. Palmoplantar keratoderma, alopecia, ectropion, and hypertrophic nails are other commonly associated findings [7]. Peripheral lymphadenopathy is common, and is defined by nodes 1.5cm or larger measured in longest traverse diameter or any palpable lymph node that is firm, irregular, clustered, or fixed [6]. However, bulky lymphadenopathy is rare at presentation. Visceral organ involvement can occur, and is associated with worse prognosis. Visceral disease has not been well defined and is likely underdiagnosed, as it may remain asymptomatic [6]. Frequent sites of visceral disease include spleen, liver, and bone marrow involvement [6]. Confirmation of involvement by biopsy of suspected organ is recommended.

Patients with SS are at increased risk for superimposed infections due to underlying immune dysfunction and physical factors such as interruption in skin barrier. Common infections include *Staphylococcus aureus*, herpes-simplex and herpes zoster, and dermatophyte infections [8]. Bacteremia and pneumonia are the major infectious causes of death in SS patients [8]. Patients with MF or SS are at an increased risk of second malignancies, most notably Hodgkin lymphoma, non-Hodgkin lymphoma, melanoma, and urinary cancers [9].

SYSTEMIC TREATMENT

There is currently no cure for SS except allogeneic stem cell transplantation. The goal of treatment is aimed at disease control and symptomatic relief [10]. Given the leukemic involvement of Sézary cells in SS, systemic treatment is typically required. A majority of patients with SS have stage III due to erythroderma (T4) or stage IV given B2 involvement in the blood. If no lymph nodes or visceral organs are involved, the stage is IVA1. The pathological presence of lymph node involvement (N3) in SS correlates with stage IVA2, whereas the presence of visceral organ involvement correlates with stage IVB.

Principles of SS Therapy

Treatment may consist of systemic therapy with or without skin-directed therapy. Skin-directed therapy may be included for symptomatic relief as reviewed in Chapter 9. Other factors affecting treatment choice include extent of disease burden, comorbid conditions, and cost [11]. There is no standard initial therapy for SS established based on randomized controlled studies. Data on treatment efficacy and outcomes is limited due to the rarity of the disease and the fact that patients with SS are often excluded from clinical trials compared to patients with MF [11]. Disease burden is defined by low-intermediate or high with a cutoff value of absolute Sézary cell count (ASC) $<$ or >5 k/μL, respectively [12].

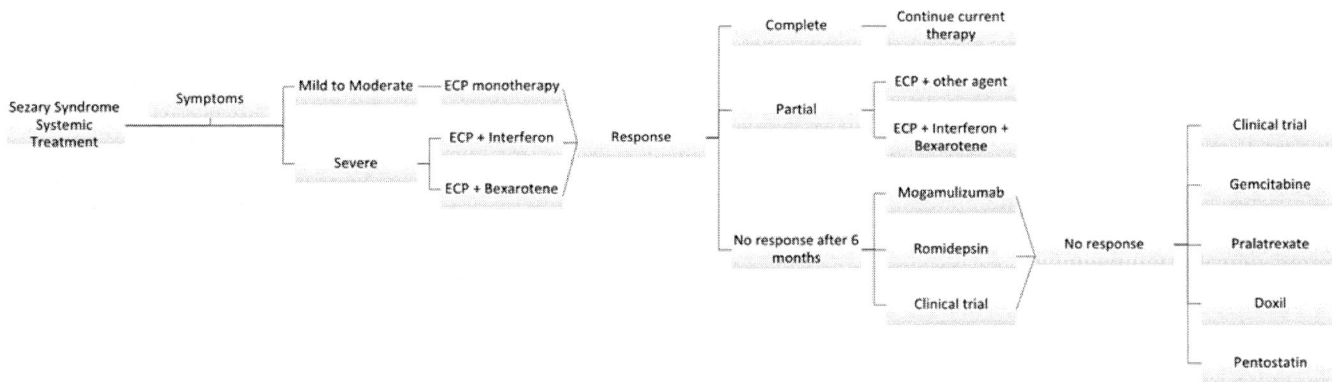

Figure 11-1. Treatment algorithm for systemic treatment for Sézary syndrome.

For low-intermediate disease burden, initial preferred regimens include monotherapy with extracorporeal photopheresis (ECP) or combinations of ECP with interferon (IFN alfa-2b or IFN gamma-1b) or retinoid (bexarotene, acitretin, isotretinoin, all-trans retinoic acid) (Fig. 11-1). Combinations of two systemic therapies are also acceptable, such as ECP plus IFN or retinoid, or all three.

Systemic regimens for relapsed/refractory low-intermediate disease burden SS include monotherapy with romidepsin, mogamulizumab, brentuximab vedotin, pralatrexate, and vorinostat. Patients with refractory disease to targeted and biological therapy can sometimes benefit from monochemotherapy such as gemcitabine, doxil or pentostatin (Fig. 11-1).

Preferred regimens for relapsed/refractory high disease burden include Mogamulizumab +/- skin directed therapy, Romidepsin +/- skin-directed therapy, or other combination therapies.

Other therapies for relapsed refractory disease include liposomal Doxorubicin, Gemcitabine, Pralatrexate, Alemtuzumab, and Pembrolizumab, Temozolamide (for CNS involvement), Bortezomib, Etoposide, and Cyclophosphamide.

Initial Therapy

Extracorporeal Photopheresis

ECP is the first FDA-approved therapy for patients with SS. ECP is a procedure involving extracorporeal separation of mononuclear cells (MNC) from peripheral blood, exposure of MNC to DNA intercalating agent 8-methoxsalen, followed by crosslinking with ultraviolet A phototherapy. This procedure induces apoptosis of malignant T-cells, activation of antigen presenting cells in the apparatus, and after subsequent infusion of MNC content back to the patient's circulation it triggers immune response against Sézary cells in blood and skin. Although time consuming, it is generally a well-tolerated procedure with minimal side effects. Treatment schedule may vary at different institutions, but is typically one or two consecutive days every 2 to 4 weeks lasting for at least 6 months. Treatment time may vary from 1.5 to 4 hours. Once maximum response achieved, a gradual taper down to once every 6 to 12 months is reasonable. Gao et al. studied the effects of 1 treatment day per week for 6 weeks, then every 2 weeks for 12 weeks, then once monthly in patients with SS or erythrodermic MF (eMF) [13]. In this retrospective study, 29/65 patients had SS. Median overall survival was 120 months for patients who underwent ECP, surpassing the historical survival range of 39-65 months [14-16]. Patients who received ECP in lines 1-3 had an improved time to next treatment (TTNT) compared to ECP used as later lines of therapy (12 versus 7 months, $p = 0.07$) [13]. TTNT was superior with ECP alone compared to IFN-alpha, bexarotene, chemotherapy, MTX, and monoclonal antibodies as monotherapy [13]. TTNT was shorter when ECP was combined with other systemic treatments [13]. Early side effects may include hypotension, fatigue, and headache. Late side effects may include mild to moderate anemia. Patients with insufficient peripheral veins may require central venous access using a specific ECP-compatible port, which may increase the risk of infection or thrombosis.

Bexarotene

Bexarotene is a systemic synthetic retinoid-X-receptor that can be used alone or in combination with skin-directed or other systemic therapy. Retinoids inhibit proliferation and induce terminal differentiation and apoptosis, although the exact mechanism in CTCL is unknown [11]. A phase II/III study in patients with SS showed an ORR of 24% with Bexarotene [17]. Side effects may include central hypothyroidism, hyperlipidemia, myelosuppression, nausea, anorexia, and teratogenicity [17].

Interferon

There are two forms of interferon alpha that are used in the treatment of SS, IFN alpha-2a and IFN alpha-2b. They differ by one amino acid; however, bind to the same receptor inducing the same effect. Pegylated forms of each are now available, which have a longer half-life. IFN as a class has cytotoxic, antiproliferative, and antiviral effects through inhibition of IL-4 and IL-5 production by T cells, thus inhibiting cytokine release [18,

19]. Resistance to IFN alpha has been observed, and is thought to be due to neutralizing antibodies, down-regulation of receptors, or lack of STAT 1 expression [11]. Overall response rates to IFN alpha in SS range from 25-50% [20-22]. IFN gamma may be used in cases of resistance to IFN alpha. IFN gamma has a similar mechanism of action, enhancing cell-mediated cytotoxicity and antiproliferation [11]. Data is limited for use in SS. Side effects to IFN alpha and gamma include flu-like symptoms such as fever, myalgias, fatigue, mild myelosuppression, hepatic transaminitis, mood changes, hypothyroidism decreased appetite, and hair thinning [11]. Side effects may be improved with acetaminophen. Side effects may be worse in the elderly and with IFN alpha compared to IFN gamma [11]. Due to discontinuation of manufacturing of IFN, these agents will likely not be available beyond 2021, unless novel agents are introduced into treatment armamentarium for patients with SS.

Therapy for Relapsed/Refractory Disease

Brentuximab Vedotin

Brentuximab vedotin (BV) is a chimeric monoclonal antibody drug conjugate that targets CD30 and is linked to monomethylauristatin E (MMAE), a micro-tubule disrupting agent. The conjugate binds to cells expressing CD30 and forms a complex which is internalized within the cell, releasing MMAE and inducing cell cycle arrest and apoptosis. In the multicenter, randomized trial (ALCANZA trial), BV was associated with superior clinical outcomes in patients with MF with CD30 expression (>10%) compared to physician's choice (ORR 65% vs 16% in MF) [23]. However, other studies showed variable responses with patients across all levels of CD30 expression. Dose-limiting toxicities include peripheral neuropathy.

Methotrexate

Methotrexate (MTX) can be used as monotherapy or in combination with other systemic or skin directed therapies. It can be given at low doses

(<100 mg/week) or intermediate doses with leucovorin rescue [24]. MTX blocks cell division in the S phase by inhibiting dihydrofolate reductase. Response rates in SS vary, ranging from 9-50% [24-27]. Potential side effects include nausea, vomiting, stomatitis, diarrhea, bone marrow suppression, liver toxicity, and pneumonitis [28]. Toxicities may be enhanced by drug interactions or underlying liver disease [28].

Mogamulizumab

Mogamulizumab is a first-in-class humanized IgG1-kappa monoclonal antibody which selectively binds to C-C chemokine receptor 4 (CCR4) with enhanced antibody-dependent cellular cytotoxicity activity [29]. CCR4 is expressed on the surface of malignant T-cells and plays a role in cell trafficking of lymphocytes into the skin [29]. The randomized phase III trial (MAVORIC trial) compared Mogamulizumab versus Vorinostat and showed superior PFS with Mogamulizumab (HR 0.32, 95% CI 0.21-0.49) in patients with SS [30]. The study showed an ORR of 37% with Mogamulizumab versus 2% with Vorinostat in relapsed/refractory SS having received at least one prior systemic treatment [30]. Of note, patients with the absence of CCR4 expression were not excluded from the trial, and clinical response did not correlate with skin expression of CCR4 [30]. The most common side effects include infusion reaction, drug rash, diarrhea, and fatigue [30]. Mogamulizumab may result in decreased number of regulatory T cells, leading to a variety of skin eruptions that may mimic CTCL but are associated with response [31]. Mild rash can be controlled with topical steroids, but more extensive and symptomatic rash usually requires treatment interruption or discontinuation.

Romidepsin

Romidepsin is an FDA-approved histone deacetylase I and II inhibitor (HDAC) used in the treatment of MF and SS. HDAC inhibitors target the epigenome and lead to alterations in chromatin structure and transcription factor activation ultimately causing cell death. Romidepsin is an intravenous HDAC inhibitor with ORR ranging from 29-35% in SS

[11, 32]. Side effects may include fatigue, nausea, decreased appetite, and EKG changes.

Vorinostat

Vorinostat is an oral HDAC inhibitor with ORR ranging from 33-36% in SS [33, 34]. Common side effects include nausea, vomiting, anorexia, fatigue. Other side effects include mild thrombocytopenia and EKG changes [11].

Doxorubicin

Doxorubicin is an anthracycline topoisomerase inhibitor used in the treatment of many other malignancies. The liposomal form allows for longer half-life. Response rates vary in CTCL, and data in SS is limited. One study noted an ORR of 66% (6 out of 9 patients) with SS [35]. Side effects may include infusion reactions, fatigue, nausea, myelosuppression, cardiac toxicity, and hand/foot syndrome [35].

Gemcitabine

Gemcitabine is a pyrimidine antimetabolite used in the treatment of many other malignancies. Most studies using Gemcitabine in SS predate the 2007 definition of SS, so response rates in CTCL range from 65-73% [11]. However, one study showed a partial response in all 11 patients treated with Gemcitabine [36]. Side effects may include fever, hypersensitivity reactions, myelosuppression, transaminitis, pneumonitis, alopecia, skin hyperpigmentation, and rarely hemolytic uremic syndrome [11].

Pralatrexate

Pralatrexate is a new anti-folate drug that has shown efficacy in MF/SS and aggressive peripheral T cell lymphomas. It is typically administered at low doses and in combination with folic acid and vitamin B12 for better side effect profile in CTCL [37]. In a dose de-escalation study, pralatrexate 15mg/m2 weekly x3 and 1 week off was found to be well tolerated. Most recently, leucovorin has been incorporated into pralatrexate regimens which significantly decreased risk of mucositis.

Alemtuzumab

Alemtuzumab is an anti-CD52 humanized IgG1-kappa monoclonal antibody that induces cytotoxicity via complement activation, antibody-dependent cellular toxicity, and direct apoptosis [38-40]. CD52 is expressed on mature, malignant B and T cells, NK cells, dendritic cells, monocytes, and eosinophils. Response rates in SS are excellent, ranging from 86-100% [41-46]. Alemtuzumab can be given intravenously or subcutaneously, and can be combined with chemotherapy [46, 47]. Lower, subcutaneous dosing improves side effect profile. Side effects may include serious and life-threatening infections including opportunistic infection and reactivation of viruses such as cytomegalovirus, herpes zoster, herpes simplex virus. Prophylactic antimicrobials are required. Other side effects include infusion reactions, myelosuppression, immune-mediated side effects, and cardiac toxicity.

Pembrolizumab

Pembrolizumab is an anti-programmed cell death 1 (PD-1) humanized IgG4 monoclonal antibody which binds to the PD-1 receptor on T cells to block the programmed cell death ligand on tumor cells from binding. This inhibits the suppression of T cell proliferation, cytokine release, and cytotoxicity by tumor cells, thus allowing the immune system to target cancer cells [48]. The CITN-10 study showed an ORR of 27% in relapsed/refractory SS [49]. Response did not correlate with PD-L1 expression on Sézary cells. Side effects include immune-mediated effects such as dermatitis, pneumonitis, diarrhea, thyroid dysfunction, hepatitis. 53% of patients treated with Pembrolizumab experienced an erythrodermic flare that did not require discontinuation of the drug, and correlated with high PD-L1 expression on Sézary cells [49].

Hematopoietic Stem Cell Transplantation

Hematopoietic stem cell transplant (HSCT) has been evaluated for the treatment of SS. Autologous HSCT is not recommended due to high relapse rates, with progression free survival (PFS) ranging from 100 days to 7 months [50]. In contrast, allogeneic HSCT in SS has shown durable remission, likely due to graft-versus-lymphoma effect. Unfortunately, high morbidity and mortality preclude many patients from this therapy. A meta-analysis comparing autologous versus allogeneic transplant in patients with relapsed/refractory MF/SS showed superior OS and EFS in the allogeneic transplant group [51]. The 5-year OS was 23% versus 80% and EFS was 0% and 60% for autologous versus allogeneic transplant, respectively [51]. Disease relapse accounted for a majority of the difference in EFS. A prospective study of 47 patients (22/47 with SS) who underwent allogeneic HSCT showed a 10.4% non-relapse mortality at 1 year, 50% relapse rate after transplant, 51% OS and 26% PFS at 4 years [52]. PFS at 4 years was superior for patients with SS compared to MF (72.7 vs 11.5, P = 0.04) [52]. Retrospective studies have reported relapse rates after allogeneic transplant to be 38-50% [53-57]. Complete remissions have been reported in patients who relapsed after transplant who received donor lymphocyte infusions, confirming graft-versus-lymphoma effect [55]. Recent advancements in allogeneic stem cell transplant have led to more favorable outcomes for patients with MF/SS, including the option of haploidentical or cord blood transplant for those with difficulty finding a matched donor, reduced intensity conditioning regimens which leads to decreased non-relapse mortality, and development of better T-cell depletion methods and immunosuppressive therapy leading to decreases in graft versus host disease (GVHD) [58]. Advanced-stage disease and unmatched donor have been shown to be poor prognostic factors for PFS after transplant [57]. Side effects of allogeneic HSCT are similar to those who undergo transplant for other diseases, including toxicities related to conditioning regimen, acute and chronic GVHD, and the need for immunosuppression post-transplant.

Future Therapies

Future therapies that are currently being evaluated for the treatment of SS include CAR-T cell therapy, bi-specific antibody therapy (BiTE) with AFM13, and IPH4102 which is a first in class anti-KIR3DL2 monoclonal antibody.

Chimeric antigen receptor modified T cell therapy (CAR-T) targeting CD30 has shown efficacy in CD30 positive lymphomas such as relapsed/refractory Hodgkin lymphoma and anaplastic large cell lymphoma [59]. A phase Ib/II trial of relapsed/refractory CD30 positive lymphoma included one patient with SS and showed a 50% ORR for the entire cohort [60]. Side effects included cytokine release syndrome. There was no evidence of neurotoxicity in either of the aforementioned trials [59, 60].

A phase I dose escalation trial of CD4 CAR-T therapy in patients with PTCL included a patient with SS who achieved CR [61]. Results of other trial patients are ongoing.

There are active CAR T/NK trials with targets such as CD3, CD4, CD5, CD7, CD30, CD37, and CCR4.

AFM13 is a CD30/CD16A bi-specific antibody that engages and activates NK cells through the activating receptor CD16 which induces antibody dependent cell mediated cytotoxicity targeting CD30 positive malignancies [62]. A phase Ib/IIa study of relapsed/refractory CD30 positive malignancies including 6/9 with MF (3/9 with systemic and cutaneous anaplastic large cell lymphoma) showed an ORR of 50% out of the entire cohort [62]. Side effects included infusion reaction.

KIR3DL2 is a cell surface protein expressed on cutaneous T cell lymphoma and Sézary cells. A phase I study of 44 patients with MF, including 35 patients with SS, treated with anti-KIR3DL2 monoclonal antibody showed an ORR of 43% in the SS cohort [63]. Side effects included fatigue, lymphopenia, and peripheral edema. A registration phase II trial, TELLOMAK, is underway to confirm efficacy in SS.

PROGNOSIS

The clinical course in SS is more aggressive than that of early stage MF. While patients may respond well to certain therapies, it is typically followed by relapse. Patients with extensive skin involvement, multiple tumors, or significant nodal or blood involvement typically have a higher risk of disease progression and decreased overall survival. Poor prognostic factors include stage IV disease, age >60, presence of folliculotropic disease in the skin, presence of large cell transformation, elevated white blood cell count, elevated LDH, and higher blood involvement of Sézary cells [64]. Disease stage as determined by TNMB staging is the strongest prognostic factor in MF/SS. Median OS for all stages of MF/SS ranges from 39-120 months [13-16, 64]. A large, multi-center, retrospective study reported a median OS of 48 and 33 months for stage IVA and IVB MF/SS, respectively [64]. Survival has improved over the last several decades as historical studies showed lower survival rates. For example, a study of a cohort of patients with SS from 1975-1997 observed a median OS of 31 months and 5 year OS of 33.5% [65]. Although MF/SS most commonly presents in older adults in the sixth to seventh decade of life, age is an important prognostic factor. MF diagnosed before age 30 has a more favorable outcome [66]. Patients with MF/SS are at increased risk of infections and secondary malignancies which contribute to decreased survival in this population. Pneumonia and bacteremia are the most common cause of death related to infection [8].

CONCLUSION

Frontline therapy for patients with SS should include extracorporeal photopheresis monotherapy or in combination with interferon or bexarotene. In the absence of response to ECP, second line therapies such as romidepsin, mogamulizumab, pralatrexate, brentuximab vedotin or vorinostst should be administered. Alemtuzumab, available only for compassionate use, can also be utilized as later line of therapy. Monochemotherapy can also be utilized in patients' refractory to targeted therapy. Even though currently available treatment options demonstrate improved survival compared to historical studies, this disease remains an unmet need, and participation in clinical trials with novel agents is recommended.

REFERENCES

[1] Sézary, A., Erythrodermie avec presence de cellules monstreuses dans derme et sang circulant. *Bull Soc Fr Dermatol Syph*, 1938. 45: p. 254-260.

[2] Bradford, P. T., et al., Cutaneous lymphoma incidence patterns in the United States: a population-based study of 3884 cases. *Blood*, 2009. 113(21): p. 5064-5073.

[3] Willemze, R., et al., WHO-EORTC classification for cutaneous lymphomas. *Blood*, 2005. 105(10): p. 3768-3785.

[4] Cristofoletti, C., M. G. Narducci, and G. Russo, Sézary Syndrome, recent biomarkers and new drugs. *Chin Clin Oncol*, 2019. 8(1): p. 2.

[5] Lamberg, S., Chairman, Mycosis Fungoides Cooperative Study Group Steering Committee: Mycosis fungoides Cooperative Study. *Arch Dermatol*, 1975. 111: p. 456-459.

[6] Olsen, E., et al., Revisions to the staging and classification of mycosis fungoides and Sézary syndrome: a proposal of the International Society for Cutaneous Lymphomas (ISCL) and the cutaneous lymphoma task force of the European Organization of Research and Treatment of Cancer (EORTC). *Blood*, 2007. 110(6): p. 1713-1722.

[7] Spicknall, K. E., Sézary syndrome-clinical and histopathologic features, differential diagnosis, and treatment. *Semin Cutan Med Surg*, 2018. 37(1): p. 18-23.

[8] Axelrod, P. I., B. Lorber, and E. C. Vonderheid, Infections complicating mycosis fungoides and Sézary syndrome. *Jama*, 1992. 267(10): p. 1354-1358.

[9] Huang, K. P., et al., Second lymphomas and other malignant neoplasms in patients with mycosis fungoides and Sézary syndrome: evidence from population-based and clinical cohorts. *Archives of dermatology*, 2007. 143(1): p. 45-50.

[10] Berg, S., et al., Multidisciplinary management of mycosis fungoides/Sézary syndrome. *Current hematologic malignancy reports*, 2017. 12(3): p. 234-243.

[11] Olsen, E. A., et al., Sézary syndrome: immunopathogenesis, literature review of therapeutic options, and recommendations for therapy by the United States Cutaneous Lymphoma Consortium (USCLC). *Journal of the American Academy of Dermatology*, 2011. 64(2): p. 352-404.

[12] Olsen, E.A., et al., Clinical end points and response criteria in mycosis fungoides and Sézary syndrome: a consensus statement of the International Society for Cutaneous Lymphomas, the United States Cutaneous Lymphoma Consortium, and the Cutaneous Lymphoma Task Force of the European Organisation for Research and Treatment of Cancer. *Journal of Clinical Oncology*, 2011. 29(18): p. 2598.

[13] Gao, C., et al., Prolonged survival with the early use of a novel extracorporeal photopheresis regimen in patients with Sézary syndrome. *Blood*, 2019. 134(16): p. 1346-1350.

[14] Fraser-Andrews, E., et al., Extracorporeal photopheresis in Sézary syndrome: no significant effect in the survival of 44 patients with a peripheral blood T-cell clone. *Archives of dermatology*, 1998. 134(8): p. 1001-1005.

[15] Sanyal, S., et al., UK national audit of extracorporeal photopheresis in cutaneous T-cell lymphoma. *The British journal of dermatology*, 2018. 178(2): p. 569-570.

[16] Siakantaris, M. P., et al., Management of cutaneous T-Cell lymphoma patients with extracorporeal photopheresis. The Hellenic experience. *Transfusion and Apheresis Science*, 2012. 46(2): p. 189-193.

[17] Duvic, M., et al., Bexarotene is effective and safe for treatment of refractory advanced-stage cutaneous T-cell lymphoma: multinational phase II-III trial results. *Journal of clinical oncology*, 2001. 19(9): p. 2456-2471.

[18] Rook, A. H. and P. Heald, The Immunopemthogenesis of Cutaneous T-cell Lymphoma. *Hematology/Oncology Clinics*, 1995. 9(5): p. 997-1010.

[19] Gottlieb, S. L., et al., Treatment of cutaneous T-cell lymphoma with extracorporeal photopheresis monotherapy and in combination with recombinant interferon alfa: a 10-year experience at a single

institution. *Journal of the American Academy of Dermatology*, 1996. 35(6): p. 946-957.

[20] Olsen, E. A. and P. A. Bunn, Interferon in the treatment of cutaneous T-cell lymphoma. *Hematology/oncology clinics of North America*, 1995. 9(5): p. 1089-1107.

[21] Papa, G., et al., Is interferon alpha in cutaneous T-cell lymphoma a treatment of choice? *British journal of haematology*, 1991. 79: p. 48-51.

[22] Jumbou, O., et al., Long-term follow-up in 51 patients with mycosis fungoides and Sézary syndrome treated by interferon-alfa. *The British journal of dermatology*, 1999. 140(3): p. 427-431.

[23] Prince, H. M., et al., Brentuximab vedotin or physician's choice in CD30-positive cutaneous T-cell lymphoma (ALCANZA): an international, open-label, randomised, phase 3, multicentre trial. *The Lancet*, 2017. 390(10094): p. 555-566.

[24] Zackheim, H. S., M. Kashani-Sabet, and S. T. Hwang, Low-dose methotrexate to treat erythrodermic cutaneous T-cell lymphoma: results in twenty-nine patients. *Journal of the American Academy of Dermatology*, 1996. 34(4): p. 626-631.

[25] Wright, J. C., et al., Observations on the use of cancer chemotherapeutic agents in patients with mycosis fungoides. *Cancer*, 1964. 17(8): p. 1045-1062.

[26] Zackheim, H. S., M. Kashani-Sabet, and A. McMillan, Low-dose methotrexate to treat mycosis fungoides: a retrospective study in 69 patients. *Journal of the American Academy of Dermatology*, 2003. 49(5): p. 873-878.

[27] Schappell, D. L., J. C. Alper, and C. J. McDonald, Treatment of advanced mycosis fungoides and Sézary syndrome with continuous infusions of methotrexate followed by fluorouracil and leucovorin rescue. *Archives of dermatology*, 1995. 131(3): p. 307-313.

[28] Olsen, E. A., The pharmacology of methotrexate. *Journal of the American Academy of Dermatology*, 1991. 25(2): p. 306-318.

[29] Ishii, T., et al., Defucosylated humanized anti-CCR4 monoclonal antibody KW-0761 as a novel immunotherapeutic agent for adult T-

cell leukemia/lymphoma. *Clinical Cancer Research*, 2010. 16(5): p. 1520-1531.

[30] Kim, Y. H., et al., Mogamulizumab versus vorinostat in previously treated cutaneous T-cell lymphoma (MAVORIC): an international, open-label, randomised, controlled phase 3 trial. *The lancet oncology*, 2018. 19(9): p. 1192-1204.

[31] Chen, L., et al., Mogamulizumab-associated cutaneous granulomatous drug eruption mimicking mycosis fungoides but possibly indicating durable clinical response. *JAMA dermatology*, 2019. 155(8): p. 968-971.

[32] Piekarz, R. L., et al., Phase II multi-institutional trial of the histone deacetylase inhibitor romidepsin as monotherapy for patients with cutaneous T-cell lymphoma. *Journal of clinical oncology*, 2009. 27(32): p. 5410.

[33] Olsen, E. A., et al., Phase IIb multicenter trial of vorinostat in patients with persistent, progressive, or treatment refractory cutaneous T-cell lymphoma. *Journal of clinical oncology*, 2007. 25(21): p. 3109-3115.

[34] Duvic, M., et al., Phase 2 trial of oral vorinostat (suberoylanilide hydroxamic acid, SAHA) for refractory cutaneous T-cell lymphoma (CTCL). *Blood*, 2007. 109(1): p. 31-39.

[35] Quereux, G., et al., Prospective multicenter study of pegylated liposomal doxorubicin treatment in patients with advanced or refractory mycosis fungoides or Sézary syndrome. *Archives of dermatology*, 2008. 144(6): p. 727-733.

[36] Duvic, M., et al., Phase II evaluation of gemcitabine monotherapy for cutaneous T-cell lymphoma. *Clinical Lymphoma and Myeloma*, 2006. 7(1): p. 51-58.

[37] Horwitz, S. M., et al., Identification of an active, well-tolerated dose of pralatrexate in patients with relapsed or refractory cutaneous T-cell lymphoma. *Blood*, 2012. 119(18): p. 4115-4122.

[38] Marcucci, G., et al., *A Novel Raji-Burkitt's Lymphoma Model for Preclinical and Mechanistic Evaluation of CD52-Targeted Immunotherapeutic Agents*.

[39] Alinari, L., et al., Alemtuzumab (Campath-1H) in the treatment of chronic lymphocytic leukemia. *Oncogene*, 2007. 26(25): p. 3644-3653.

[40] Nückel, H., et al., Alemtuzumab induces enhanced apoptosis in vitro in B-cells from patients with chronic lymphocytic leukemia by antibody-dependent cellular cytotoxicity. *European journal of pharmacology*, 2005. 514(2-3): p. 217-224.

[41] Kennedy, G., et al., Treatment of patients with advanced mycosis fungoides and Sézary syndrome with alemtuzumab. *European journal of haematology*, 2003. 71(4): p. 250-256.

[42] Lenihan, D. J., et al., Cardiac toxicity of alemtuzumab in patients with mycosis fungoides/Sézary syndrome. *Blood*, 2004. 104(3): p. 655-658.

[43] Zinzani, P. L., et al., Preliminary observations of a phase II study of reduced-dose alemtuzumab treatment in patients with pretreated T-cell lymphoma. *Haematologica*, 2005. 90(5): p. 702-703.

[44] Gautschi, O., et al., Successful treatment of chemotherapy-refractory Sézary syndrome with alemtuzumab (Campath-1H). *European journal of haematology*, 2004. 72(1): p. 61-63.

[45] Querfeld, C., et al., Alemtuzumab for relapsed and refractory erythrodermic cutaneous T-cell lymphoma: a single institution experience from the Robert H. Lurie Comprehensive Cancer Center. *Leukemia & lymphoma*, 2009. 50(12): p. 1969-1976.

[46] Alinari, L., et al., Subcutaneous alemtuzumab for Sézary Syndrome in the very elderly. *Leukemia research*, 2008. 32(8): p. 1299-1303.

[47] Porcu, P., et al., Phase I trial of subcutaneous (SQ) alemtuzumab (A) and CHOP in T-cell lymphoma: preliminary results. *Journal of Clinical Oncology*, 2006. 24(18_suppl): p. 7594-7594.

[48] Robert, C., et al., Anti-programmed-death-receptor-1 treatment with pembrolizumab in ipilimumab-refractory advanced melanoma: a randomised dose-comparison cohort of a phase 1 trial. *The Lancet*, 2014. 384(9948): p. 1109-1117.

[49] Khodadoust, M.S., et al., Pembrolizumab in relapsed and refractory mycosis fungoides and Sézary syndrome: a multicenter phase II study. *Journal of Clinical Oncology*, 2020. 38(1): p. 20.

[50] Duarte, R., et al., Haematopoietic stem cell transplantation for patients with primary cutaneous T-cell lymphoma. *Bone marrow transplantation*, 2008. 41(7): p. 597-604.

[51] Wu, P. A., et al., A meta-analysis of patients receiving allogeneic or autologous hematopoietic stem cell transplant in mycosis fungoides and Sézary syndrome. *Biology of Blood and Marrow Transplantation*, 2009. 15(8): p. 982-990.

[52] Hosing, C., et al., Allogeneic stem-cell transplantation in patients with cutaneous lymphoma: updated results from a single institution. *Annals of Oncology*, 2015. 26(12): p. 2490-2495.

[53] Schlaak, M., et al., Allogeneic stem cell transplantation for advanced primary cutaneous T-cell lymphoma: a systematic review. *Critical reviews in oncology/hematology*, 2013. 85(1): p. 21-31.

[54] de Masson, A., et al., Allogeneic stem cell transplantation for advanced cutaneous T-cell lymphomas: a study from the French Society of Bone Marrow Transplantation and French Study Group on Cutaneous Lymphomas. *haematologica*, 2014. 99(3): p. 527.

[55] Iqbal, M., et al., Efficacy of allogeneic hematopoietic cell transplantation in cutaneous T cell lymphoma: results of a systematic review and meta-analysis. *Biology of Blood and Marrow Transplantation*, 2020. 26(1): p. 76-82.

[56] Lechowicz, M. J., et al., Allogeneic hematopoietic cell transplantation for mycosis fungoides and Sézary syndrome. *Bone marrow transplantation*, 2014. 49(11): p. 1360-1365.

[57] Domingo-Domenech, E., et al., Allogeneic hematopoietic stem cell transplantation for advanced mycosis fungoides and Sézary syndrome. An updated experience of the Lymphoma Working Party of the European Society for Blood and Marrow Transplantation. *Bone Marrow Transplantation*, 2021: p. 1-11.

[58] Johnson, W.T., et al., Allogeneic hematopoietic stem cell transplantation in advanced stage mycosis fungoides and Sézary syndrome: a concise review. *Chinese clinical oncology*, 2018. 8(1): p. 12-12.

[59] Ramos, C.A., et al., Clinical and immunological responses after CD30-specific chimeric antigen receptor–redirected lymphocytes. *The Journal of clinical investigation*, 2017. 127(9): p. 3462-3471.

[60] Grover, N.S., et al., Clinical responses to CAR. CD30-T cells in patients with CD30+ lymphomas relapsed after multiple treatments including brentuximab vedotin. *Blood*, 2018. 132(Supplement 1): p. 681-681.

[61] Zhang, H., et al., *First-in-Human CD4 CAR Clinical Trial on Peripheral T-Cell Lymphoma*. 2019, American Society of Hematology Washington, DC.

[62] Sawas, A., et al., Clinical and Biological Evaluation of the Novel CD30/CD16A Tetravalent Bispecific Antibody (AFM13) in *Relapsed or Refractory CD30-Positive Lymphoma with Cutaneous Presentation: A Biomarker Phase Ib/IIa Study* (NCT03192202). Blood, 2018. 132(Supplement 1): p. 2908-2908.

[63] Bagot, M., et al., IPH4102, a first-in-class anti-KIR3DL2 monoclonal antibody, in patients with relapsed or refractory cutaneous T-cell lymphoma: an international, first-in-human, open-label, phase 1 trial. *The Lancet Oncology*, 2019. 20(8): p. 1160-1170.

[64] Scarisbrick, J. J., et al., Cutaneous Lymphoma International Consortium study of outcome in advanced stages of mycosis fungoides and Sézary syndrome: effect of specific prognostic markers on survival and development of a prognostic model. *Journal of Clinical Oncology*, 2015. 33(32): p. 3766.

[65] Bernengo, M. G., et al., Prognostic factors in Sézary syndrome: a multivariate analysis of clinical, haematological and immunological features. *Annals of oncology*, 1998. 9(8): p. 857-863.

[66] Crowley, J. J., et al., Mycosis fungoides in young patients: clinical characteristics and outcome. *Journal of the American Academy of Dermatology*, 1998. 38(5): p. 696-701.

In: Mycosis Fungoides and Sézary Syndrome ISBN: 978-1-68507-093-9
Editors: X. Zhang and L. Sokol

Chapter 12

Pathogenesis and Diagnosis of Sézary Syndrome

Hailing Zhang**, MD
Department of Pathology,
H. Lee Moffitt Cancer Center and Research Institute,
Tampa, FL, USA

Introduction

Sézary Syndrome (SS) is a rare aggressive leukemic variant of cutaneous T cell lymphoma (CTCL) and is closely related to mycosis fungoides (MF). It is a disease of older adults, more prevalent in males, with an average disease onset of 50-60 years [1]. The frequency of SS is globally stable at 3% of CTCL [2]. Clinically, SS is known to carry an aggressive clinical course with 5-year overall survival ranges between 10% and 30% (depending on ISCL and EORTC clinical stage), and median survival is approximately 30 months [3]. SS is originally defined by the triad of exfoliative erythroderma (erythema involving more than 80% of the skin

* Corresponding Author's Email: hailing.zhang@moffitt.org.

surface), generalized lymphadenopathy, and clonally related neoplastic T cells with cerebriform nuclei (Sézary cells) in the skin, lymph nodes, and peripheral blood. More recently, WHO 2017 classification of lymphoid malignancies [3] illustrated additional criteria for blood involvement: either an absolute Sézary cell count ≥ 1,000/μL or an expanded CD4+ T-cell population resulting in a CD4:CD8 ratio ≥ 10, CD4+/CD7- cells ≥ 40%, or CD4+/CD26- cells ≥ 30% of the lesional lymphocytes.

Clinically, erythroderma is a characteristic sign of SS, in which the entire skin becomes red with intense pruritus, and sometimes edema and scaling, particularly on the palms and soles. Hepatomegaly, alopecia, ectropion, and nail dystrophy are common manifestations, and generalized lymphadenopathy is often present [4]. In the end-stage of the disease, all visceral organs may be involved. SS cases are more likely to have a shorter duration of onset compared to MF. However, there are occasions of SS arising in patients with long-standing MF that progresses slowly. The ISCL recommends that such cases be designated as "SS preceded by MF." Conversely, patients with MF, but without erythroderma, may meet hematologic criteria for SS. In these cases, the designation "MF with leukemic involvement" is recommended [5]. In addition to erythroderma, other clinical features in SS include alopecia (scalp and/or other body areas), ectropion (eversion of eyelids and exposure of conjunctiva), palmoplantar scaling/keratoderma. There are no known risk factors for SS.

Sézary cells are considered to have different cell of origin when compared with MF by phenotype and molecular signatures. Expression of CD3, CD4, CD45RO, and CCR4 indicates a mature memory T-cell phenotype, and expression of CCR7, L-selectin, and CD27 suggests skin-tropic central memory T-cell. Sézary cells also express T-regulatory profile (CD25 and FOX-P3) phenotypes, which result in suppression of the immune response [6]. In contrast, the phenotype seen in MF cells is consistent with skin resident memory T-cells.

Table 12-1. Staging according to International Society of Cutaneous Lymphomas (ISCL)/European Organization for Research and Treatment of Cancer (EORTC) system

Stage		T	N	M	B	Median OS (Years)	5 Year OS [a] (%)	5 Year DSS (%)
Early	IA	1	0	0	0–1			
		Limited patches or plaques <10% skin surface	No nodal involvement	No visceral involvement	<1000 atypical cells	35.5	N/S	98
	IB	2	0	0	0–1			
		Patches or plaques ≥10% skin surface	No nodal involvement	No visceral involvement	<1000 atypical cells	21.5	86	89
	IIA	1–2	1–2	0	0–1			
		Any patches or plaques	Aggregates of atypical cells	No visceral involvement	<1000 atypical cells	15.8	N/S	89
Advanced	IIB	3	0–2	0	0–1			
		Tumoral lesions	No involvement or aggregates of atypical cells	No visceral involvement	<1000 atypical cells	4.7	62	56
	III	4	0–2	0	0–1			
		Erythroderma	No involvement or aggregates of atypical cells	No visceral involvement	<1000 atypical cells	4.7	N/S	56
	IIIA	4	0–2	0	0			
		Erythroderma	No involvement or aggregates of atypical cells	No visceral involvement	<250 atypical cells	4.7	60	54
	IIIB	4	0–2	0	1			
		Erythroderma	No involvement or aggregates of atypical cells	No visceral involvement	250–1000 atypical cells	3.4	54	48
	IVA_1	1–4	0–2	0	2			
		Any skin involvement	No involvement or aggregates of atypical cells	No visceral involvement	>1000 atypical cells + clonality	3.8	52	41
	IVA_2	1–4	3	0	0–2			
		Any skin involvement	Partial or complete effacement of nodal architecture	No visceral involvement	<1000 or >1000 atypical cells + clonality	2.1	34	23
	IVB	1–4	0–3	1	0–2			
		Any skin involvement	Any nodal involvement	Visceral involvement	<1000 or >1000 atypical cells + clonality	1.4	23	18

STAGING

Staging of MF and SS is based on TNMB system (skin, lymph node, visceral involvement and completed with blood involvement) and revised according to International Society of Cutaneous Lymphomas (ISCL)/European Organization for Research and Treatment of Cancer (EORTC) system (Table 12-1) [7].

SS patients are erythrodermic (T4) with peripheral blood involvement ranges from B0 to B2: Stage B0 cases have < 250 atypical cells (CD4 + CD7 − or CD4 + CD26 −) and represents no significant blood involvement, as identified by flow cytometry; Stage B1 cases contain 250 – 1000 atypical cells and represent low blood tumor burden; Stage B2 features ≥ 1000 atypical cells and high blood tumor burden [8]. Bone marrow involvement is generally not considered in this staging system.

PATHOLOGIC FEATURES

SS can be a challenge to diagnose especially in the early phase due to broad clinical differential diagnosis and because skin biopsies can be non-specific in up to one-third of otherwise classic SS cases [9]. Definitive skin biopsies in SS patients will show similar histologic features of MF: atypical lymphocytic infiltrate with epidermotropism, the classic "Pautrier microabscesses" and sometimes "large cell transformation." There may be a dense bandlike lymphocytic infiltrate. The lymphocytes are monotonous and atypical with epidermotropism. However, epidermotropism is often less prominent and can be absent. Up to one third of SS skin biopsies may be non-diagnostic showing non-specific fidings, even with prominent spongiosis [9]. Therefore, the patient with suspicious SS should be thoroughly assessed including peripheral blood flow cytometry and T cell gene clonality studies.

When the SS diagnosis is made only by biopsies of the involved lymph nodes and/or by examination of peripheral blood circulating Sézary cells, additional helpful tools include the demonstration of consistent T cells receptor clonality in skin/lymph nodes biopsies and peripheral blood through molecular studies.

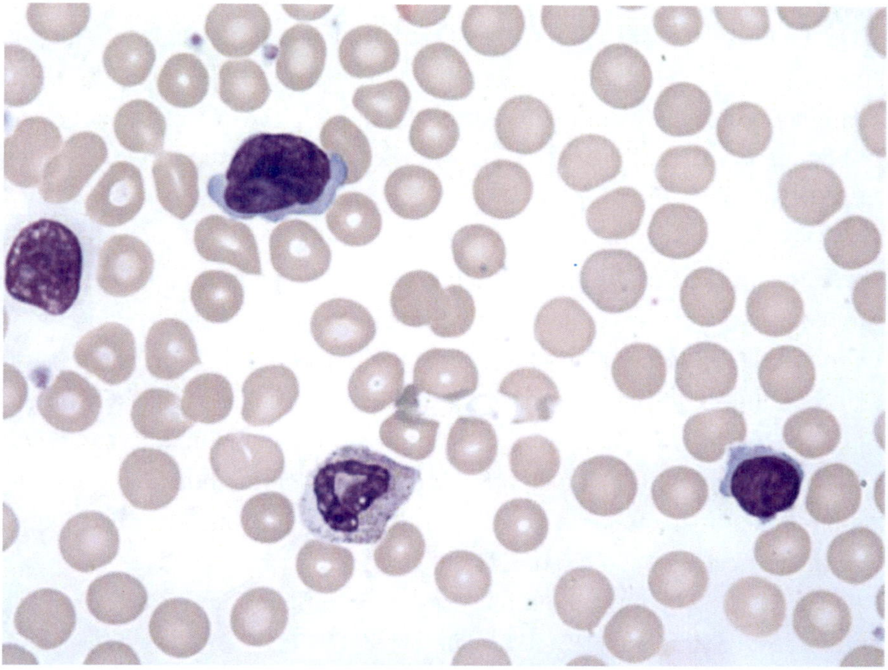

Figure 12-1. Sézary cell show typical cerebriform nuclei. Background neutrophil and lymphocyte can be seen (courtesy of Dr. Ling Zhang, H. Lee Moffitt Cancer Center).

The classic morphologic findings in involved lymph nodes include effacement of the normal lymph node architecture by dense infiltrate of atypical lymphoid cells (Sézary cells). These atypical lymphoid cells are usually monotonous comparing to other peripheral T cell lymphomas. The Sézary cell count in peripheral blood is crutial for SS diagnosis. Sézary cells by morphology is defined by circulating atypical lymphocytes with hyperchromatic, convoluted ceribriform nuclei (Fig. 12-1). Currently morphologic examination for detection and quantification of Sézary cells has largely been replaced by multiparameter flow cytometry because of a high interobserver variability in cell counts, and the fact that atypical lymphocytes with cerebriform nuclei can be found in PB from healthy people and patients with reactive conditions [10, 80-82]. Furthermore, a small cell variant of the Sézary cell has been described and these neoplastic cells whould not have been detected morphologically [11].

By flow cytometry, the neoplastic cells are generally positive for CD2, CD3, CD5 and TCRβ, and mostly CD4. They can rarely be CD8+. Aberrant loss of CD7 can be observed in two third of the cases, while CD2, CD3 and CD5 can be lost as well. It should be noted that CD7 loss can also be seen in benign dermatoses. Loss of CD26 can be seen in the majority of the cases [12-16].

This diagnosing and staging method of evaluating CD4 + CD7- or CD4 + CD26- by ISCL/EORTC can be problematic since normal CD4+ T-cells almost always contain a subset of cells with no/weaker CD26 and/or CD7 expression. These numbers may further increase in reactive/inflammatory skin conditions [17]. More recently, the International Clinical Cytometry Society (ICCS) reached a consensus to characterize and enumerate MF/SS cells based on multiparameter flow cytometric immunophenotyping for immunophenotypical aberrancy, rather than a simple, individual evaluation and quantification of CD26 or CD7-negative cells [18].

The ICCS recommendation uses a minimum combination of six antibodies, including CD3, CD4, CD8, CD7, CD26, and CD45. This simple combination could detect most aberrant MF/SS CD4+ T-cells discriminated from background normal T-cells. In addition to loss of CD7 and CD26, aberrantly dim to complete loss of surface expression of CD3 can be seen in 40-80% of blood involvement by MF/SS. Slight dim expression of CD4 and altered expression of light scatter can be seen in up to 50% of cases. It is also important to include CD8 in the panel to exclude CD4/CD8 double-positive T cells, which can be seen in many reactive conditions. Finally, a CD4:CD8 ratio is known to have important diagnostic and prognostic value and has been included in WHO 2017 diagnostic criteria.

Additional antigens mentioned in ICCS recommendations that could have a potential contribution to the detection of Sézary cells include CD2, CD5, CD164, CD158k, CD194 (CCR4), CD279 (PD-1), CD10, CD45RO, and CD38. However, utilization of these antigens should depend on the combination of at least CD3, CD4, CD7 and CD26 in the same analysis tube and the final interpretation needs to be cautioned with extensive validation and consultation. Sézary cells are typically positive for CD279, CCR4 and CD52, negative for CD30. They should be expected to be mostly positive or slightly dim for CD2 and CD5, almost always positive for TCRαβ, negative for TCRγδ, CD56 and CD57.

Furthermore, there is an emerging utilization of T-cell receptor constant β chain-1 (TRBC1) expression by flow cytometric in the diagnosis of T-cell malignancies including Sézary syndrome [19]. This is an antibody specific for one of two mutually exclusive TRBC1 expression showing promise for a rapid confirmation of clonality in immunophenotypically aberrant T-cells [20].

Molecular studies, including detection of a clonal TCR gene rearrangement by PCR and the presence of a clonal cytogenetic abnormality, provide evidence of T-cell clonality. Alternatively, Vβ repertoire analysis has been shown to be able to confirm clonality in suspected T cell lymphoproliferative disorders with immunophenotypic aberrancies [21]. However, Vβ repertoire analysis is costly and the test faces the same limitation as the PCR-based T cell gene rearrangement studies.

As mentioned before, the identification and quantification of Sézary cells have been moved away from manual count to the utilization of flow cytometry. The ICCS guideline strongly recommends quantifying tumor burden by the composite flow cytometry immunophenotyping, not to use CD26 negative or CD7 negative CD4 positive cells as surrogates of SS/MF cells. The absolute Sézary cell enumeration can be done using a single flow cytometric assay, or more commonly, by the calculation from a percentage of Sézary cell determined by flow cytometry and CBC data from hematology analyzer.

GENETIC AND MOLECULAR ALTERATIONS

Similar to advanced MF patients, diverse and complex genomic abnormalities are commonly seen in SS. The findings include chromosomal aberrations most often involving losses of 1p, 6q, 10q and gains of 8q and

17q, among others [22]. None of these chromosomal abnormalities is found in the ponderance of cases. Overall, somatic copy number variations (SCNVs) are favored over single nucleotide variants (SNVs). High throughput sequencing techniques revealed a heterogeneous novel gene mutation pattern indicating chromosomal instability because of abnormal DNA repair machinery, activation of RAG endonucleases, impaired cell cycle control, and widespread DNA hypomethylation [23]. Recent NGS studies also revealed frequent mutations in elements of pathways related to DNA damage repair (*TP53*), apoptosis (*FAS*), cell cycle (*MYC*, *RB1*), epigenetic modulators (*DNMT3A*, *TET2*), JAK/STAT (*JAK3, STAT3, STAT5B*), *ARID1A, NFKB2, CARD11*, TCR-signaling (*CD28, PLCG1*) [23, 24]. Most point mutations are C >T because of age-related and UVB-related mutagenesis.

SS has been traditionally considered to be an leukemic phase of MF. However, recent studies revealed phenotypic and genetic differences between MF and SS, suggesting that the two diseases derive from different sets of memory T cells [25] and have different molecular pathogenesis, and therefore warrant distinct therapeutic strategies [26, 27]. Sézary cells appear to be derived from central memory T cells, which express lymph node homing molecules CCR7 and L-selectin as well as the differentiation marker CD27. In contrast, neoplastic T cells isolated from MF skin lesions lacked CCR7, L-selectin and CD27 but strongly expressed CCR4 and CLA, a phenotype suggestive of origion of effector memory T cells [25]. Supportive to this finding, cytokine production profiles differ between MF and SS as well [28]. Recent studies also show that recurrent chromosomal alterations in MF markedly differ from that observed in SS [22, 27, 29]. Some of the somatic mutations revealed by NGS in multiple pathways are also found in MF [30].

Differential Diagnosis Condideration

There are many inflammatory conditions that can cause erythroderma and many of these conditions can simulate SS clinically and pathologically.

The diagnosis of SS must be established with great caution, best with a clinician together. The most common causes of erythroderma include psoriasis, pityriasis rubra pilaris, generalized allergic contact dermatitis, and drug eruptions. Pathlogically, the skin biopsies of these erythrodermic inflammatory conditions should comply with the underlying condition.

TREATMENT

Patients with SS often require a multidisciplinary approach, with combinations of skin-directed therapies, biologic-response modifiers and systemic chemotherapy. A "risk-adapted" stage-based approach, consistent with NCCN guidelines, is adopted, with biologic-response modifiers (e.g., bexarotene and interferon-alpha) and histone deacetylase. Although recognized by NCCN, these therapies often fail to provide durable responses. Targeted therapies have variable response rates ranging from 30% to 67%, with complete responses no higher than 41% [31]. In addition, nonmyeloablative allogeneic stem cell transplantation, the only potential cure for advanced MF/SS, has a 46% OS at 5 years [32]. Complete remission status before the transplantation is an important predictor for the successuful treatment. Due to the limited efficacy of the SS treatments, patients are often encougred to participate in available clinical trials.

SUMMARY

In summary, SS is often a challenging diagnosis to make due to broard clinical differential diagnosis, non-specific skin biopsy findings and difficulties in peripheral blood atypical lymphocyte phenotyping. In addition to thorough clinical examination, classic MF histology on skin biopsies, peripheral blood examination with multiparameter flow cytometry and T cell receptor gene rearrangement studies on both skin and blood specimens are critical for correct diagnosis and staging. The recent ICCS recommended to quantify MF/SS by enumerating immunophenotypically aberrant CD4+ T-cells, rather than CD26− or CD7− in isolation. This method allows to distinguish MF/SS cells from background benign T-cells and enables for more accurate staging.

References

[1] Willemze, R., et al. The 2018 update of the WHO-EORTC classification for primary cutaneous lymphomas. *Blood*, 2019. 133(16): p. 1703-1714.

[2] Dobos, G., et al. Epidemiology of Cutaneous T-Cell Lymphomas: A Systematic Review and Meta-Analysis of 16,953 Patients. *Cancers* (Basel), 2020. 12(10).

[3] Swerdlow, S., et al. *WHO classification of Tumours of Haematopoietic and lymphoid tissues*. 4th (revision) ed. 2017, Lyon, France: IARC.

[4] Goodlad, J. and E. Calonje, *Cutaneous lymphoproliferative diseases and related disorders.*, in McKee's pathology of the skin: with clinical correlations, E. Calonje, et al., Editors. 2012, Elsevier/Saunders: Edinburgh.

[5] Hristov, A. C., T. Tejasvi, and R. A. Wilcox, Mycosis fungoides and Sézary syndrome: 2019 update on diagnosis, risk-stratification, and management. *Am. J. Hematol.*, 2019. 94(9): p. 1027-1041.

[6] Spicknall, K. E., Sézary syndrome-clinical and histopathologic features, differential diagnosis, and treatment. *Semin. Cutan. Med. Surg.*, 2018. 37(1): p. 18-23.

[7] Olsen, E., et al. Revisions to the staging and classification of mycosis fungoides and Sézary syndrome: a proposal of the International Society for Cutaneous Lymphomas (ISCL) and the cutaneous lymphoma task force of the European Organization of Research and Treatment of Cancer (EORTC). *Blood*, 2007. 110(6): p. 1713-22.

[8] Garcia-Diaz, N., et al. Mycosis Fungoides and Sézary Syndrome: An Integrative Review of the Pathophysiology, Molecular Drivers, and Targeted Therapy. *Cancers* (Basel), 2021. 13(8).

[9] Trotter, M. J., et al. Cutaneous histopathology of Sézary syndrome: a study of 41 cases with a proven circulating T-cell clone. *J. Cutan. Pathol.*, 1997. 24(5): p. 286-91.

[10] Jawed, S. I., et al. Primary cutaneous T-cell lymphoma (mycosis fungoides and Sézary syndrome): part I. Diagnosis: clinical and histopathologic features and new molecular and biologic markers. *J. Am. Acad. Dermatol.*, 2014. 70(2): p. 205 e1-16; quiz 221-2.

[11] Lutzner, M. A., et al. Cytogenetic, cytophotometric, and ultrastructural study of large cerebriform cells of the Sézary syndrome and description of a small-cell variant. *J. Natl. Cancer Inst.*, 1973. 50(5): p. 1145-62.

[12] Wilcox, R. A., Cutaneous T-cell lymphoma: 2014 update on diagnosis, risk-stratification, and management. *Am. J. Hematol.*, 2014. 89(8): p. 837-51.

[13] Bogen, S. A., et al. Immunophenotypic identification of Sézary cells in peripheral blood. *Am. J. Clin. Pathol.*, 1996. 106(6): p. 739-48.

[14] Hristov, A. C., E. C. Vonderheid, and M. J. Borowitz, Simplified flow cytometric assessment in mycosis fungoides and Sézary syndrome. *Am. J. Clin. Pathol.*, 2011. 136(6): p. 944-53.

[15] Sokolowska-Wojdylo, M., et al. Absence of CD26 expression on skin-homing CLA+ CD4+ T lymphocytes in peripheral blood is a highly sensitive marker for early diagnosis and therapeutic monitoring of patients with Sézary syndrome. *Clin. Exp. Dermatol.*, 2005. 30(6): p. 702-6.

[16] Pierson, D. M., et al. Utility of CD26 in flow cytometric immunophenotyping of T-cell lymphomas in tissue and body fluid specimens. *Cytometry B Clin. Cytom.*, 2008. 74(6): p. 341-8.

[17] Boonk, S. E., et al. Evaluation of Immunophenotypic and Molecular Biomarkers for Sézary Syndrome Using Standard Operating Procedures: A Multicenter Study of 59 Patients. *J. Invest. Dermatol.*, 2016. 136(7): p. 1364-1372.

[18] Horna, P., et al. Flow cytometric evaluation of peripheral blood for suspected Sézary syndrome or mycosis fungoides: International

guidelines for assay characteristics. *Cytometry B Clin. Cytom.*, 2021. 100(2): p. 142-155.

[19] Horna, P., et al. Emerging Role of T-cell Receptor Constant beta Chain-1 (TRBC1) Expression in the Flow Cytometric Diagnosis of T-cell Malignancies. *Int. J. Mol. Sci.*, 2021. 22(4).

[20] Shi, M., et al. Single Antibody Detection of T-Cell Receptor alphabeta Clonality by Flow Cytometry Rapidly Identifies Mature T-Cell Neoplasms and Monotypic Small CD8-Positive Subsets of Uncertain Significance. *Cytometry B Clin. Cytom.*, 2020. 98(1): p. 99-107.

[21] Gibson, J. F., et al. Cutaneous T-cell lymphoma (CTCL): Current practices in blood assessment and the utility of T-cell receptor (TCR)-Vbeta chain restriction. *J. Am. Acad. Dermatol.*, 2016. 74(5): p. 870-7.

[22] Vermeer, M. H., et al. Novel and highly recurrent chromosomal alterations in Sézary syndrome. *Cancer Res.*, 2008. 68(8): p. 2689-98.

[23] Choi, J., et al. Genomic landscape of cutaneous T cell lymphoma. *Nat. Genet.*, 2015. 47(9): p. 1011-9.

[24] Woollard, W. J., et al. Candidate driver genes involved in genome maintenance and DNA repair in Sézary syndrome. *Blood*, 2016. 127(26): p. 3387-97.

[25] Campbell, J. J., et al. Sézary syndrome and mycosis fungoides arise from distinct T-cell subsets: a biologic rationale for their distinct clinical behaviors. *Blood*, 2010. 116(5): p. 767-71.

[26] LeBoit, P. and L. Pincus, *Mycosis fungoides and Sézary syndrome.*, in Hematopathology, E. Jaffe, et al., Editors. 2016, Elsevier: Philadelphia, PA. p. 713-729.

[27] van Doorn, R., et al. Oncogenomic analysis of mycosis fungoides reveals major differences with Sézary syndrome. *Blood*, 2009. 113(1): p. 127-36.

[28] Saed, G., et al. Mycosis fungoides exhibits a Th1-type cell-mediated cytokine profile whereas Sézary syndrome expresses a Th2-type profile. *J. Invest. Dermatol.*, 1994. 103(1): p. 29-33.

[29] Mao, X., et al. Molecular cytogenetic analysis of cutaneous T-cell lymphomas: identification of common genetic alterations in Sézary

syndrome and mycosis fungoides. *Br. J. Dermatol.*, 2002. 147(3): p. 464-75.

[30] da Silva Almeida, A. C., et al. The mutational landscape of cutaneous T cell lymphoma and Sézary syndrome. *Nat. Genet.*, 2015. 47(12): p. 1465-70.

[31] Trautinger, F., et al. European Organisation for Research and Treatment of Cancer consensus recommendations for the treatment of mycosis fungoides/Sézary syndrome - Update 2017. *Eur. J. Cancer,* 2017. 77: p. 57-74.

[32] Duarte, R. F., et al. Long-term outcome of allogeneic hematopoietic cell transplantation for patients with mycosis fungoides and Sézary syndrome: a European society for blood and marrow transplantation lymphoma working party extended analysis. *J. Clin. Oncol.*, 2014. 32(29): p. 3347-8.

ABOUT THE EDITORS

Xiaohui Zhang, MD, PhD

Associate Member, Department of Pathology
H. Lee Moffitt Cancer Center and Research Institute, Tampa, FL, USA
(ORCID ID: 0000-0002-1033-7550)
Email: Xiaohui.Zhang@moffitt.org

Dr. Xiaohui Zhang is a hematopathologist at H. Lee Moffitt Cancer Center, Tampa, FL. His clinical focus is in hematopathology, including leukemia, lymphoma and other hematologic disorders. He has been in a cutaneous T cell lymphoma workgroup for many years and works closely with the CTCL clinical and research teams.

Lubomir Sokol, MD, PhD

Senior member, Department of Malignant Hematology,
H. Lee Moffitt Cancer Center and Research Institute, Tampa, FL, USA
(ORCID ID: 0000-0003-0916-547X)
Email: Lubomir.Sokol@moffitt.org

Dr. Lubomir Sokol is a senior hematologist/oncologist at H. Lee Moffitt Cancer Center, Tampa, FL. His clinical and laboratory work has been focused on T-cell lymphomas/leukemias and he has been the Co-Director of the Cutaneous Lymphoma Multidisciplinary Clinic for over 15 years. This clinic is the largest referral center for patients with cutaneous T cell lymphoma in the southeastern U.S.

INDEX

A

B

C

D

E

F

G

H

I

J

K

L

M

N

O

P

R

S

T

U

V

W

X

Y

Z